Super Smoothies

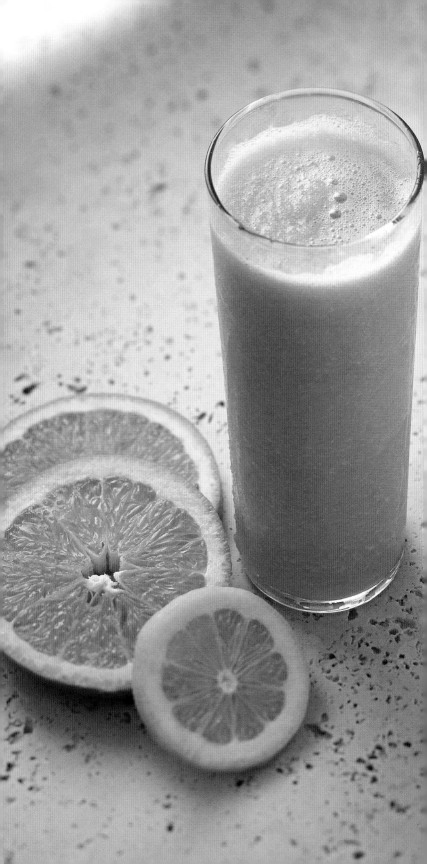

Super Smoothies

100 Recipes to Supercharge Your Immune System

Ellen Brown
with Karen Konopelski, M.S., R.D.

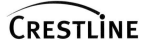

This edition published in 2013 by
CRESTLINE
an imprint of BOOK SALES
a division of Quarto Publishing Group USA INC.
142 West 36th Street, 4th Floor
New York, New York 10018
USA

This edition published by arrangement with Fair Winds Press, a member of
Quayside Publishing Group, 100 Cummings Center, Suite 406L Beverly, MA 01915

First published in the USA in 2009 by Fair Winds Press as *Supercharge Your Immune
System*

Text © 2008 Fair Winds Press

10 9 8 7 6 5

Library of Congress Cataloging-in-Publication Data
Brown, Ellen.
  Supercharge your immune system : 100 ways to help your body fight illness, one
glass at a time / Ellen Brown.
      p. cm.
  Includes index.
  ISBN 978-0-7858-3006-1
  1. Smoothies (Beverages) 2. Blenders (Cookery) 3. Immunity—Nutritional aspects.
  4. Autoimmune diseases—Nutritional aspects. I. Title.
  TX840.B5B763 2008
  641.5'63—dc22

                                                    2007038950

Book design by Liz Trovato
Photography by Glenn Scott Photography

Printed and bound in China
Reprinted 2013, 2014 twice, 2015

The information in this book is for educational purposes only. It is not intended to
replace the advice of a physician or medical practitioner. Please see your health
care provider before beginning any new health program.

This book is dedicated to
Ilan, Mira, and Lev Dubler-Furman,
the small folk who bring such large joy to my life.

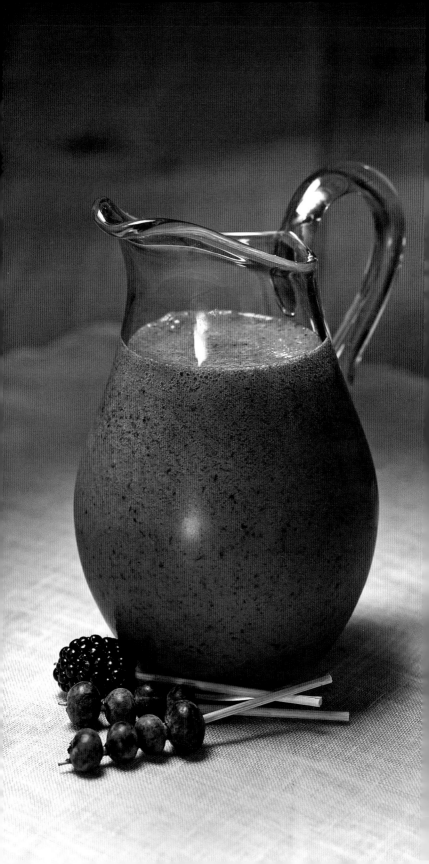

CONTENTS

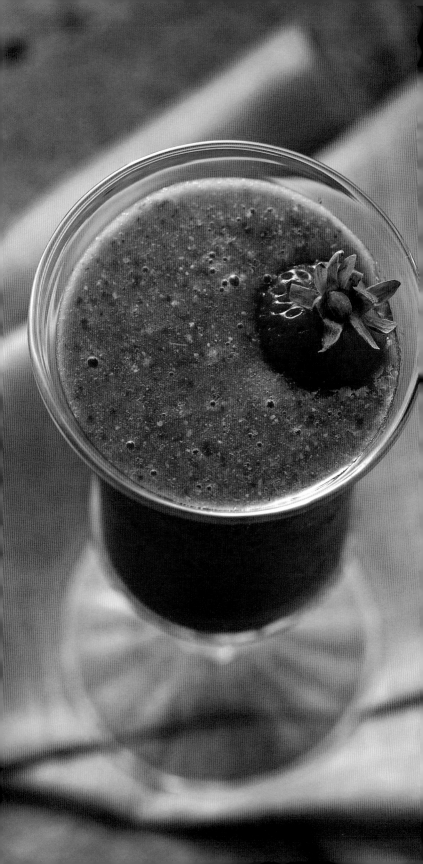

PREFACE

There has been something of a nutritional awakening in the past decade, and we now fully appreciate the direct correlation between our diet and overall health. We now know what foods are bad for our health and can lead to problems ranging from heart disease to cancer, and we also know what foods promote good health by delivering key nutrients that the body cannot make and therefore must obtain from either foods or pills containing nutritional supplements.

Cutting back on the so-called "bad fats"—first saturated fat and then trans fat—while increasing the variety and amounts of fruits, vegetables, and whole grains we eat daily has become part of our way of life. These foods now form the base of the nutritional pyramid that has replaced the former food groups chart.

For many people, however, a dichotomy exists between the centerpieces of our meals and what we eat for snacks or dessert. These treats may not be filled with empty calories from refined sugar or processed grains, but neither are they contributing to our health and well-being—and they should be.

Smoothies fill the niche when you want a food that tastes decadent during the day or at the end of a meal, but you also want it to be good for you. Smoothies are the healthful grandchildren of the malteds and milkshakes of my youth, and they can be created from a cornucopia of nutritious fruits and other beneficial ingredients. For breakfast they are the perfect "car cuisine" because they can be sipped while driving. They are a flavorful treat for children and adults at any time of day, and they make wonderful desserts, too.

The smoothies in *Super Smoothies* accomplish much more than quenching your thirst with thick and frosty drinks. I chose specific ingredients that contain the nutrients you need to keep your all-important immune system in optimal condition. The immune system has a vital role in protecting your body from disease and fighting infection if it does invade.

It is an interesting paradox that as modern medicine has eradicated many of the diseases that were potentially fatal in past eras, the current levels of environmental pollutants threaten our immune systems on a daily basis. Rather than the immune system having less work these days, it is tested every time we breathe.

Each of these one hundred recipes is annotated both for its overall nutritional content and for the specific nutrients it delivers that fortify the immune system. But we don't sip numbers; we sip smoothies. And these recipes are designed to tempt your taste buds and give you the satisfaction of a decadent treat.

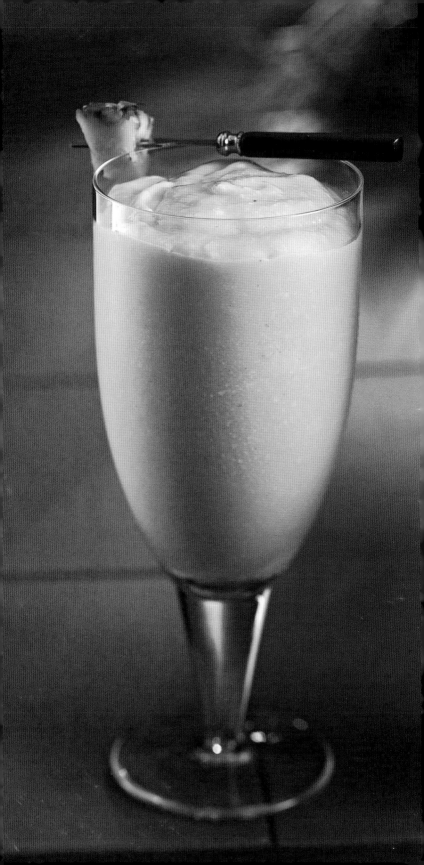

CHAPTER 1
THE FOOD PHARMACY: HOW NUTRIENTS KEEP YOU HEALTHY

Adages such as "An apple a day keeps the doctor away" and "You are what you eat" are true: There is a direct correlation between a diet rich in nutrients and low in fat and our ability to remain healthy. A crucial component of good health is a strong immune system that guards against penetration by harmful micro-organisms and fights them if they manage to infect the body.

We are now able to identify which nutrients boost our immune system, making it possible to prime that valuable pump and keep it in top form. This chapter is a crash course of the immune system that will introduce you to its multiple facets. You'll also learn which nutrients are vital for keeping this defense system as robust as possible.

HOW YOUR IMMUNE SYSTEM PROTECTS YOU FROM HARM

The immune system is a collection of complementary defense mechanisms that protects against infection by identifying and killing pathogens—any outside invader that triggers an immune response—that can range from viruses and bacteria to parasites and fungi. It is not easy for the immune system to detect these pathogens: They want to survive so they have a way of adapting to the host organism—in this case your body—in an effort to remain undetected. The immune system must therefore act like a well-trained commando; it is trained to look beneath the camouflage, find the pathogen, and then destroy it.

Every living organism—including those with a single cell—is armed with this type of defense mechanism. However, in highly developed species like humans, this mechanism has evolved into a complex system made up of many types of proteins, cells, organs, and tissues that interact as a dynamic network.

The immune system protects you from infection with layered defenses of increasing specificity. First there are physical barriers—termed nonspecific defenses—that prevent pathogens from entering the body. The most obvious physical barrier is your tough outer covering of skin and membranes. As long as the skin remains free of injuries ranging from scrapes and burns to irritation from chemicals, it can hold the body's insides in and safely keep the rest of the world out.

Other barriers protect the internal parts of your body that are open to pathogens. Enzymes in the mouth's saliva and nose hairs, for example, are part of the immune system, and involuntary acts such as coughing and sneezing eject pathogens from your respiratory tract.

In your stomach, gastric acid serves as a chemical defense against pathogens. Other bodily fluids also form part of this first line of defense. Tears flush out your eyes, and urine expels pathogens from the urinary tract.

If pathogens or toxins make it past the nonspecific defenses, specific defenses (described later in this chapter) are activated. For the immune system to work properly, two things must happen: Your body must recognize that it has been invaded, and the immune response must be activated quickly before the pathogens gain a strong hold.

The Organs That Keep You Healthy

As we now know, the immune system is a complex and dynamic network that battles to keep infection out of our bodies and fight it if it penetrates. While all components of the immune system work harmoniously to battle diseases, some are more vital than others. For example, we can live without our tonsils and spleen but not without our skin or bone marrow.

The organs involved with the immune system are called lymphoid organs and their functioning—along with that of the lymphatic vessels— makes up the lymphatic system. The lymphoid organs work together to produce infection-fighting white blood cells called lymphocytes, which are released into the bloodstream and play a vital role in keeping us healthy.

The lymphatic system has three related functions: It removes excess fluids from body tissues, it absorbs fatty acids, and it transports these needed fatty acids to the circulatory system. The system is comprised of the following:

- **Lymph nodes.** Small organs (they range in size from a few millimeters to a centimeter) shaped like kidney beans with a honeycomb structure, lymph nodes are located throughout the body and connect with one another via the lymphatic vessels. They are sometimes incorrectly called lymph glands; however, they are not glands because they do not secrete substances. The five hundred to six hundred nodes in our bodies have clusters in the underarms, groin, neck, chest, and abdomen. These nodes are components of the lymphatic system, and they contain white blood cells and filter foreign particles. These nodes swell when the body is fighting an infection due to their accumulation of lymphocytes and fluid.
- **Lymphatic vessels.** A network of channels that carry the lymphocytes to the organs and into the bloodstream, the lymphatic system, in contrast to the blood system, is not closed and has no central pump

such as your heart. Its movement is slow and has low pressure due to peristalsis—smooth muscle contractions of the intestinal tract—and the slow squeezing (called a "milking action") of skeletal muscles. Like veins, however, lymphocytes travel through vessels in one direction only.

- **The spleen.** An organ about the size of a small fist, it is located in the upper left part of the abdominal cavity behind the stomach and just below the diaphragm. It is held in place by ligaments to other organs such as the stomach and kidney. The spleen acts like a filter. It destroys old red blood cells and filters the blood that captures foreign materials.
- **The thymus.** An organ comprised of two lobes that are joined by strands of connective tissue, it is located above the heart and below the thyroid gland. Each lobe is organized into two compartments: The cortex is the outer compartment and the medulla is the inner compartment. Lymphocytes divide in the cortex, and, as the T-cells mature, they migrate into the medulla and eventually into the bloodstream. Although the thymus gland becomes vestigial by the onset of puberty, it plays a critical role in the development of a child's immune system both before birth and during the first two years of life.
- **Adenoids.** Two glands located at the back of the nasal passage, where the nose blends into the mouth, their function—like that of all lymphoid tissue—is to trap infectious agents and produce antibodies. Due to their position, they most often defend against pathogens that are inhaled into the body.
- **The tonsils.** Two ovals at the back of the throat, their position allows them to defend against upper respiratory tract infections. Both adenoids and tonsils are frequently removed, especially in children, due to their propensity for infection. In the event they are surgically removed, other components of the immune system work harder to fill the gap.
- **The blood vessels,** which include arteries and veins through which blood flows. If laid end to end, the blood vessels in an average human body would stretch more than sixty thousand miles.
- **Bone marrow.** The spongy tissue found inside the cavities of our bones, bone marrow initially produces all blood cells—white blood cells (leukocytes), red blood cells (erythrocytes), and platelets (thrombocytes)—through a process called hematopoiesis. There are two types of bone marrow, red and yellow, and the lighter color is due to a much higher number of fat cells. The red marrow is found mainly in flat bones, like the hips and shoulder blades, and the yellow marrow is found in the hollow interior of the middle portion of long bones.

Why Cells Are Your Soldiers

All blood cells, including lymphocytes, are produced from stem cells within the bone marrow. If they continue to mature in the bone marrow, they become B-cells, while other lymphocytes complete maturation in the thymus and become T-cells. These two groups of cells recognize when infectious micro-organisms have infiltrated the body and begin to attack them.

The first step is that these cells sense the presence of an antigen (a foreign substance that invades the body), which stimulates an immune response. The word antigen was coined because it stimulates *anti*body *gene*ration. Some antigens enter the body from the outside; we may inhale them or ingest them in food. These antigens frequently trigger allergic reactions. Other antigens are generated within the cells as a result of normal cell metabolism or because of viral or bacterial infection.

B-cells give rise to cells that produce proteins called antibodies and secrete them into the body's fluids. Antibodies can bind to the antigen and interfere with its ability to function. Alternatively, they can stimulate an inflammatory response that attracts neutrophils, monocytes, and macrophages (types of white blood cells) to the site of infection and kills the bacteria in one of two ways: by penetrating the cell's membrane or by activating a complementary antigen that targets the first antigen for attack as it would a healthy cell (the two antigens basically neutralize each other). B-cells are free to circulate in the bloodstream, but they cannot penetrate living tissue.

T-cells work in a different way. The major difference is that they are created as immature cells and are sent to the thymus to be programmed to recognize one specific target antigen. A T-cell can move anywhere in the body, and it can destroy cells that it has been programmed to attack by attaching itself to the targeted cell and injecting it with strong chemicals.

T-cells are divided into two groups. "Killer T-cells" destroy cells that have been infected with viruses and other pathogens or are otherwise damaged; this type of cell is very important in blocking the replication of viruses. "Helper T-cells" regulate the immune responses by communicating with other cells, and they help determine what type of immune response the body will make to a specific pathogen (think of them as traffic cops). T-cells can assist B-cells by triggering a chain reaction that causes the B-cell to form plasma cells. These plasma cells then begin to produce more B-cells, thus allowing the number of antibodies to increase exponentially. Other T-cells then have the job of monitoring the level of antigens present in the body, and they will stop the production of B-cells when the infection has been eliminated.

While these are the two main types of cells, there are others. Granulocytes or polymorphonuclear (PMN) leukocytes are another group of white blood cells whose primary importance is removing bacteria and parasites from the body. They engulf these foreign bodies and degrade them using powerful enzymes.

Macrophages are scavenger cells that help initiate and regulate the immune response. They pick up and ingest antigens and present these foreign materials to the B-cells and T-cells for destruction.

Another cell type, dendritic cells, originates in the bone marrow and functions in a similar way. They are usually found in the lymphoid organs, although they can be in the bloodstream or other tissues of the body. Dendritic cells capture antigens and bring them to one of the lymphoid organs to trigger an immune response.

HOW WE RID OURSELVES OF INVADERS

Now that you know all the players, here is a summary of how the game is played, or, in this case, how an immune response works. The membrane of virtually every cell is studded with various proteins, which together are known as the major histocompatibility complex, or MHC. The MHC molecules function as transporters, carrying fragments of proteins from within the cell to the cell surface, where they are presented to the immune system. T-cells only recognize an antigen if it is carried on the surface of a cell by one of the body's own MHC molecules.

The scouts then begin. The first action is that a macrophage or dendritic cell—called the antigen-presenting cell, or APC—begins working in combination with either a B-cell or a T-cell. If the APC presents an antigen on its surface to a B-cell, the B-cell is signaled to proliferate and produce antibodies that specifically bind to the antigen. These antibodies then destroy the antigen. If the APC presents the antigen to a T-cell, the T-cell is activated to kill the antigen.

Battling Free Radicals with Antioxidants

The role of oxygen in our lives is a mixed blessing: It's essential to maintain life, yet it simultaneously harms our cells. To put it in the simplest terms, an antioxidant is a substance in the diet that reduces cellular damage that has been caused by oxygen.

When molecules anywhere in the body are afflicted by oxygen, they are called free radicals. Unfortunately, we don't have a magic bullet to prevent molecules from becoming free radicals because it is a natural part of the metabolic process. Moreover, environmental pollution has increased the number of free radicals in our bodies, and we therefore have a greater need for antioxidants.

The cell damage caused by free radicals can lead to anything from heart disease to cancer, so mitigating their effects with antioxidants is crucial to your health. Even skin creams are now formulated with antioxidant nutrients to counteract the effects of ultraviolet light, one of the environmental causes of cell damage.

We now know that maintaining a diet rich in antioxidants—found in fresh fruits and vegetables—is a way to boost the immune system. Many of the protective functions of the immune cells depend on the fluidity of the membranes of the cell. Free radicals reduce this fluidity and keep the cells of the immune system from their appointed tasks.

A bit of chemistry is necessary to understand how antioxidants and free radicals interact. The human body is composed of many different types of cells, and cells are composed of many different types of molecules. Molecules consist of one or more atoms of one or more elements joined by chemical bonds.

As you probably remember from science class, atoms consist of a nucleus, neutrons, protons, and electrons. The protons—positively charged particles—are located in the atom's nucleus while the electrons—negatively charged particles—surround the atom. Electrons orbit an atom in one or more shells, and the most important structural feature in determining the chemical behavior of an atom is the number of electrons in its outer shells. A substance with a full outer shell is inert, but an atom will try to fill its outer shell by gaining or losing electrons or by sharing its electrons by bonding together with other atoms.

Normally, bonds do not split in a way that leaves a molecule with an odd, unpaired electron. But when weak bonds split, free radicals are formed. These free radicals begin to attack the nearest stable molecule to capture the electron needed to gain stability. This triggers a chain reaction: When the "attacked" molecule loses its electron, it, too, becomes a free radical. Antioxidants are known as "free radical scavengers"—they neutralize free radicals by donating one of their own electrons, thus ending the electron "stealing" action.

Antioxidant nutrients do not become free radicals themselves when they donate electrons because they are stable in either form. So they roam the body and act like a good housekeeper, mopping up free radicals before they can inflict damage on cells and tissue. For example, the cholesterol in your body is not harmful until it becomes oxidized, at which point it begins to cling to your blood vessels and clog your arteries, possibly leading to heart disease and stroke.

Many antioxidants work best when combined because they contain complementary nutrients; in this case, the whole is greater than the sum of its parts. And drinking smoothies offers you a significant advantage because they typically contain complementary antioxidants.

HOW TO USE FUNCTIONAL FOODS FOR HEALTH

Your immune system is the body's first line of defense against bacteria, viruses, and other foreign invaders. However, the immune system can only fight infection if it is constantly supplied with the necessary "weapons." Foods are the crucial supply lines that support the troops.

With rare exception—such as our ability to generate vitamin D when exposed to sunlight—eating foods that are high in specific immune-boosting nutrients is the best way for our bodies to gain access to these key disease fighters. The body needs protein, fatty acids, vitamins, and minerals on a daily basis. Ideally these nutrients should come from the foods we eat; the alternative is to take vitamin and mineral supplements.

Vitamins are either water soluble or fat soluble, and those that are water soluble cannot be stored in the body for more than a brief amount of time before they are removed by the kidneys and excreted in the urine. The entire group of B vitamins, including the immune-boosting B6 and antioxidant-loaded vitamin C, fall into this group.

Fat-soluble vitamins are absorbed using bile acids (the fluids used to digest fats). Once they are absorbed, your body stores them in the liver and body fat and removes them when necessary. The fat-soluble vitamins that matter most to the immune system are vitamin A and vitamin E.

While it is possible to identify the exact levels of vitamins in the foods we eat, the mineral content will vary depending on a number of factors. This is because minerals come from the earth or from water, and plants and animals absorb them to get nutrients. The mineral content of the food is therefore dependent on: the mineral content of the soil in which the food was grown; the minerals present in the water used for irrigation or nourishment by the animal food source; and the mineral content of the foods eaten by the animal food source. Magnesium, manganese, selenium, copper, iron, and zinc are the minerals most closely linked to a strong immune system.

It is preferable to obtain vitamins and minerals from food rather than from a pill because nutrients must be taken in tandem for the body to achieve optimal benefits and supplement pills do not contain the same phytonutrients as foods. For example, iron absorption is increased when it is taken with vitamin C, and vitamin D aids in the absorption of calcium (the reason most milk is fortified with vitamin D).

In the past decade the international nutritional community has begun to advocate a diet that goes beyond simply maintaining a healthy immune system to one that actively aids in the prevention of disease and enables the immune system to fight disease if it occurs. A study published by the *European Journal of Clinical Nutrition* refers to this diet as "functional food," which is the term used by countries in the European Union; in the United States the term "nutraceutical" is frequently used.

Functional foods are conventional foods eaten as part of a normal diet that contain large amounts of immunity-boosting nutrients. All of the smoothie recipes in this book were formulated with ingredients that qualify as functional foods. The advantage of eating them as part of a smoothie is that you accomplish the primary goal of combining foods with complementary nutrients—easily and deliciously.

HOW NUTRIENTS BOOST
YOUR IMMUNE SYSTEM

Every five years, the U.S. Department of Health and Human Services joins forces with the U.S. Department of Agriculture to advise Americans on ways to promote health and prevent disease. In 2005, the date of the most recent report, they found that many Americans consume more calories than they need without meeting the recommended intakes for a number of key nutrients. These nutrients include:

- For adults: calcium, potassium, fiber, magnesium, and vitamins A, C, and E.
- For children and adolescents: calcium, potassium, fiber, magnesium, and vitamin E.

An additional premise of the federal dietary guidelines is that these nutrients should come primarily from foods that are termed "nutrient dense," meaning foods that provide substantial amounts of vitamins and minerals and relatively few calories. The reason it is important to gain these nutrients from foods rather than supplements is that foods also contain hundreds of naturally occurring substances, including carotenoids and flavonoids, that may protect against chronic health conditions. You will find all of the listed nutrients in the fruits, nuts, and other ingredients used in this book's smoothie recipes, in addition to protein and carbohydrates, which the body also needs to function properly.

Super-Star Nutrients

Certain nutrients play a more pivotal role in boosting the immune system than others. Here are the most important nutrients for keeping your immune system in tip-top shape and for boosting it when necessary to fight illness:

- **Carotenoids**—Beta-carotene, which gives foods like carrots, sweet potatoes, peaches, and papayas their orange color, may be the member of this group you read the most about, but there are many others in this widespread category of naturally occurring pigments. All carotenoids provide what is termed provitamin A, which the body converts to retinol, the active form of vitamin A. Lycopene, which gives tomatoes their red color, is a carotenoid that has been widely discussed by the news media for its role in preventing heart disease. (Because lycopene operates slightly differently from the majority of the pigment-producing compounds, it is discussed separately later.) Carotenoids are powerful antioxidants and therefore enhance the functioning of the immune system. Luckily, there is a veritable rainbow of fruits that are high in these valuable nutrients.
- **Copper**—Two delicious smoothie ingredients, sesame seeds and sunflower seeds, are particularly high in this mineral. Copper is an essen-

tial component of many enzymes, so it plays a role in many physiological processes. Most of the copper content in your bloodstream is incorporated into a compound called ceruloplasmin, an enzyme that facilitates the oxidation of minerals, including iron.

- **Cysteine**—Many smoothie recipes include yogurt—in part because of its cysteine content. Cysteine is an amino acid that protects cells from free radical damage. It also breaks down proteins found in mucous that settles in the lungs, making it very helpful to the respiratory system.

- **Flavonoids**—This term encompasses more than six thousand different substances that are found in plants and are responsible for their color. Most flavonoids function in your body as antioxidants and regulate inflammation—your body's natural response to danger—so that the immune system is not overly stimulated. The final benefit of flavonoids to your immune system is that they can act as an antibiotic by disrupting the progress of certain viruses or bacteria (this antiviral action has proven effective with the herpes simplex virus, for example).

- **Folate**—Your immune system's first line of defense is the skin, and that's where folate becomes important. Folate is a B-complex vitamin most recognized for its importance during pregnancy in preventing birth defects, but its significance is far more wide ranging. Folate helps to produce and maintain new skin cells, and it is needed to make DNA and RNA, the building blocks of cells.

- **Glutamine**—Your body synthesizes this amino acid from another amino acid called glutamic acid or glutamate. In addition to supporting the health of your intestinal tract, glutamine helps to maintain the body's acid-base balance. Glutamine is pertinent to your immune system because it serves as a precursor (a chemical that is transformed into another compound) to the antioxidant glutathione.

- **Iron**—Sustaining a proper level of this mineral is crucial because iron serves as the core of the hemoglobin molecule, which is the oxygen-carrying component of red blood cells. Its role in the immune system is a general one, but a good supply of dietary iron helps optimize blood iron levels.

- **Lipoic acid**—This nutrient is vital to your body because it helps turn glucose (blood sugar) into energy for the body's needs. Lipoic acid is the only antioxidant that can deactivate free radicals in both water-based and fat-based environments. As an antioxidant, lipoic acid prevents oxygen-based damage to nerves, and it has also been shown to strengthen the effects of other antioxidants such as vitamins C and E.

- **Lycopene**—A member of the carotenoid family of phytonutrients, lycopene is most often associated with the red color of tomatoes, although it is found in foods as diverse as watermelon and peanuts. Unlike several of its carotenoid cousins, lycopene does not get converted into vitamin A, so its health benefits flow from its powerful antioxidant actions. Lycopene is also believed to play a role in the prevention of heart disease by inhibiting free radical damage to LDL cholesterol. Before cholesterol can be deposited in the plaques that harden and narrow arteries, it must be oxidized by free radicals. With its powerful antioxidant activity, lycopene can prevent LDL cholesterol from being oxidized.

- **Magnesium**—Like all minerals, magnesium cannot be made in our body and must therefore be plentiful in our diet. Many chemical reactions in the body involve the presence of enzymes, which are special proteins that help trigger chemical reactions. More than three hundred different enzymes in the body require magnesium in order to function. Magnesium is also involved in carbohydrate metabolism to release energy when we need it and protein synthesis as cells build proteins.

- **Manganese**—This mineral is both essential and potentially toxic (if taken in sufficiently large quantities). It plays a central role in a number of physiologic processes as a constituent of certain enzymes and as an activator of others. Manganese is part of the principal antioxidant enzyme in the mitochondria (the cell's power producers). And because the mitochondria consume more than 90 percent of the oxygen used by the cells, they are especially vulnerable to oxidative stress.

- **Omega-3 fatty acids**—Recent reports that omega-3 fatty acids could be an important defense against anything and everything from cardiovascular disease to depression and rheumatoid arthritis elevated oily fish like salmon to the top of people's list of essential foods. Since these polyunsaturated fats (also found in nuts and flaxseeds) help prevent disease, they should be considered vital to a healthy immune system. The cells in your body are surrounded by a membrane composed primarily of fatty acids, and it is through the cell membrane that nutrients enter the cell and waste products are removed from the cell. The omega-3 fatty acids in the cell membranes have been shown to activate an enzyme that suppresses tumor growth. Additionally, omega-3 fatty acids increase the activity of phagocytes, which are the white blood cells that eat up bacteria.

- **Potassium**—Like magnesium, potassium is a background player in boosting your immunity, and you need a proper level of it in your body so that components of the immune system are free to fight infection. Along with sodium and chloride, potassium is a member of the electrolyte family of minerals. Potassium is important for keeping your muscles and nerves functioning properly and for maintaining an appropriate acid-base balance in your body.

- **Protein**—Proteins are complex molecules made up of a combination of different amino acids, which, in turn, are compounds containing a number of various chemical elements. Amino acids are divided into essential—those the body cannot make on its own and must come from diet—and nonessential—those the body can make, though it is still more efficient for the body to gain them from food because food contains a much higher level than the body can produce. Protein is a chief source of energy for the body, providing four calories per gram. In the complicated workings of the immune system, proteins are necessary for the production of antibodies. Antibodies are proteins that attach themselves to antigens (viruses, bacteria, or other foreign forces) and deactivate them so they can be destroyed.

- **Selenium**—This micro-mineral is needed on a daily basis in your diet but only in very small amounts; in fact the amount in foods is measured in micrograms, which are one thousandth of a milligram. While a food's mineral content depends on the soil in which it is grown, selenium seems particularly sensitive to variations in soil. The primary purpose of selenium in the immune system is to protect cells against oxidative damage. To do this the selenium works with a group of nutrients—including vitamins C and E—to prevent oxygen molecules from becoming overly reactive. Selenium also prevents DNA damage, thereby inhibiting the multiplication of cancer cells.

- **Vitamin A**—A fat-soluble vitamin, vitamin A is frequently referred to as the "anti-infective" vitamin thanks to its role in maintaining a healthy immune system. Preformed vitamin A can be found in foods of animal origin like eggs and milk. Your body also converts the carotenoids found in many fruits and vegetables into vitamin A. This vitamin enhances the operation of white blood cells, increases the response of antibodies to danger, and also has an antiviral function. In addition, vitamin A helps maintain healthy skin and mucous membranes, which are the immune system's first line of defense.

- **Vitamin B6**—Enzymes are the proteins that help chemical reactions take place in your body, and vitamin B6 is involved in more than one hundred enzymatic reactions. It is difficult to find a category of molecules in your body that does not depend in some way on vitamin B6. Many of the building blocks of protein, called amino acids, require adequate supplies of B6 for synthesis, and vitamin B6 plays a role in all new cell formation. This vitamin also has a hand in processing carbohydrates when your body needs energy.

- **Vitamin C**—British sailors became known as "limeys" in the eighteenth century because they discovered that eating limes—an excellent source of vitamin C—prevented scurvy, a disease of the gums and skin. Also called ascorbic acid, vitamin C is powerful enough to prevent fruits such as apples or avocados from browning, and prevention is the same role it plays in your immune system. This water-soluble nutrient must be consumed on a regular basis (any excess is excreted from the body), and since humans are one of the few animal species that cannot make vitamin C, it is essential to take in a sufficient amount on a regular basis. Vitamin C operates in your immune system as a powerful antioxidant and prevents oxygen-based damage to cells. Vitamin C also prevents cell damage in lipids, which are the fats and oils in our bodies.

- **Vitamin E**—This fat-soluble vitamin is actually an entire family that exists in eight different forms. Its importance lies in preventing a condition called oxidative stress from developing in your cells. Vitamin E works with vitamin C, selenium, and other nutrients to keep the oxygen molecules from becoming too reactive and damaging the cell structures around them.

- **Zinc**—Like copper and manganese, zinc is a micro-mineral that we need on a daily basis but only in a small amount. Zinc's functions include building DNA and RNA inside the nucleus of cells and keeping blood sugar levels and metabolic rates even. In the immune system, zinc is important to the functioning of lymphocytes. A deficiency of zinc can diminish both the number of these crucial white blood cells and their response to antigens.

ABOUT AUTOIMMUNE DISORDERS

It would seem logical that if you feed your immune system the proper nutrients at sufficient levels on a regular basis, then all should be well. Unfortunately, for people with autoimmune disorders it's not that simple. These diseases can turn the immune system upside down.

At any given time your body is filled with billions of B-cells and T-cells that are programmed to find a specific antigen and destroy it. However, in some cases, a cell is created that does not follow its protocol. Rather than targeting and destroying the intruding antigen, such as a virus or bacteria, the cell attacks the body's healthy cells and tissues.

This can happen in a few ways. In some cases, the B-cells go awry and produce antibodies that attach themselves to cells that are not harmful. These antibodies then start to multiply and kill off some of the "good cells." On the T-cell side, a malfunction within the thymus is the trigger. Occasionally the thymus fails to provide accurate programming for T-cells and they are given a genetic code of an organ tissue or other cell that your body needs to function. These wrongly-programmed T-cells then attach themselves to healthy tissue and begin to destroy it.

There are more than eighty types of autoimmune disease, and many of them share similar symptoms. For example, lupus and rheumatoid arthritis—two of the more common autoimmune diseases—both cause joint pain and stiffness. With lupus, swelling and damage to the joints, skin, blood vessels, and organs occurs. With rheumatoid arthritis, inflammation begins in the tissues lining the joints and spreads to the entire joint, resulting in muscle pain, weakness, and deformed joints.

Other types of autoimmune diseases damage only a single organ or tissue; Hashimoto's thyroiditis, for example, involves an underactive thyroid gland, while Graves' disease is the result of an overactive thyroid. Celiac disease, Crohn's disease, and ulcerative colitis, on the other hand, all affect the gastrointestinal tract.

While autoimmune disorders are not yet fully understood, some causes are now accepted by many medical authorities. The sources of these disorders include: viruses that change the information carried inside the cells; sunlight and other forms of radiation; and certain chemicals and drugs. There is also an apparent link to sex hormones, as many more women than men suffer from autoimmune disorders.

At the present time there are no cures for autoimmune diseases, but keeping a healthy immune system can mitigate some of the debilitating symptoms. That is where the smoothies in this book can be of help; the recipes are formulated to boost the immune system with key nutrients.

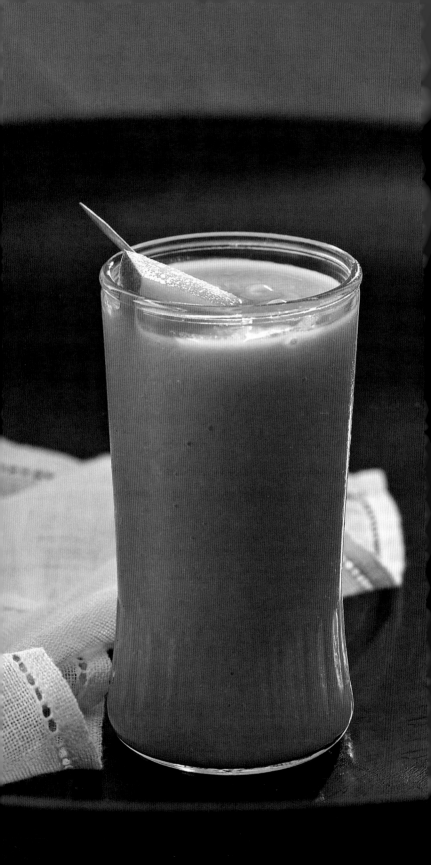

CHAPTER 2
FOODS TO SUPERCHARGE YOU

Here's a wonderful reality: eating luscious fruits can actually make you healthier by building your immune system! And while there is no such thing as a fruit that is bad for you, some are richer than others in the nutrients you need to boost immunity. In this chapter you will learn about these fruits and the nutrients they contain. Once you understand the basics, you can start improvising your own smoothie recipes.

You will notice that most of the recipes in this book contain more ingredients than just fruit or fruit products. These "supporting player" ingredients range from dairy products like yogurt to soy-based tofu to certain powders and other nutritional enhancements, such as flaxseed oil (which is rich in omega-3 fatty acids). These bonus ingredients add flavor and texture to the smoothie while contributing their own high nutritional values to the mix.

THE IMPORTANCE OF ORGANICS

Both for your body and for the planet, it is essential to use organic ingredients whenever possible. The term "organic" was somewhat vague until 2001, when the U.S. Department of Agriculture set standards that clearly defined the meaning of the word, both in terms of food and farming practices.

Organic agriculture prohibits the use of most synthetic fertilizers and pesticides, sewer sludge fertilizers, genetic engineering, growth hormones, irradiation, antibiotics, and artificial ingredients. The antioxidants in our bodies have to work even harder today to combat the ravages of environmental pollutants, and organic farming does its part by taking a stand against pollution.

When you see meats, eggs, or dairy products carrying the organic label, you know that the animals have not been given drugs or growth hormones, and they have been kept in conditions that allow for regular exercise and humane treatment.

In terms of saving the Earth, the agricultural practices used for organic farming are environmentally friendly. Soil fertility and crop nutrient management must be conducted in a way that improves soil conditions, minimizes erosion, and prevents crop contamination. Farmers must use crop rotation methods and fertilize with composted animal manure and plant materials rather than chemicals. Pests are controlled by traps rather than chemical sprays, and plastic mulches are forbidden.

THE HEAVY HITTERS

Each of the ingredients in these smoothie recipes has been selected for a specific reason: They contain a high proportion of the nutrients and phytonutrients necessary to keep your immune system pumped up and primed to fight free radicals and ward off infection.

These are the fruits and other ingredients you will find most often in super smoothies:

Fruits and a Few Veggies

- **Apples**—Flavonoids are the nutrient stars of apples; the skin is an excellent source of quercitin, which is a very potent flavonoid. Moreover, a 100-gram serving (one small apple or approximately one cup of slices) provides approximately 16 percent of your daily vitamin C needs (100 grams of apple has about 9 milligrams of vitamin C). Of all the fruits used in these smoothie recipes, apples deliver the greatest concentration of flavonoids. Flavonoids are a subset of polyphenols, which are a group of phytonutrients that are powerful antioxidants; it is the flavonoids that give fruits and vegetables their vibrant colors. The flavonoids from an apple contain about 22 percent of the polyphenols consumed by the average American in the course of a day, and they are more readily absorbed into the bloodstream than polyphenols gained from other foods. (Note: cloudy apple juice has more nutrients than clear apple juice.)
- **Apricots**—Both in their fresh and dried form, succulent apricots are a boon to your immune system, delivering a hefty amount of vitamin A. They also contain lycopene, a potent antioxidant.
- **Avocados**—Like bananas, avocados add a creamy texture to smoothies without using a dairy product, and their buttery richness allows them to blend well with both fruits and vegetables. They are an excellent source of vitamin K—which is necessary for proper blood clotting—in addition to potassium, folate, and dietary fiber.
- **Bananas**—You will find a number of smoothie recipes, in this book and others, that list bananas as an ingredient. This is because their texture acts as a binder to emulsify the smoothie without asserting a strong taste. Bananas are a treasure trove of vitamin B6, are high in potassium, and low in sodium.
- **Blackberries**—Like blueberries, blackberries are an excellent source of flavonoids. They are also a very good source of vitamin C, dietary fiber, and manganese, and they contain vitamin E, folate, and magnesium.

- **Blueberries**—A Tufts University study showed that blueberries are the fruit with the highest antioxidant activity, and a whole cup has just eighty calories. These berries are a terrific source of vitamin C, and their blue-red pigment is packed with photonutrients known as anthocyanidins that neutralize damage caused by free radicals.
- **Cantaloupe**—A cantaloupe's bright orange color should be a tip-off that this low-calorie fruit—a one-cup serving contains a mere fifty-six calories—is loaded with beta-carotene. In addition, a one-cup serving delivers more than 100 percent of the Daily Value or DV (the recommended amount of a nutrient eaten on a daily basis) for vitamin A and vitamin C. Cantaloupe is also a good source of potassium, vitamin B6, and folate.
- **Carrots**—This root vegetable is equally good when added to smoothies or when its sweet flavor and moisture are added to carrot cake. One medium carrot provides more than twice your daily requirement of vitamin A (a one-cup serving of carrots contains more than 400 percent of the DV). Carrots are also a good source of vitamins C and K and potassium.
- **Cranberries**—It is now more than a decade since the American Medical Association gave scientific validity to the widely held belief that cranberry juice reduces the risk of urinary tract infections. Cranberries do so because they contain an antibacterial agent called hippuric acid, which reduces the ability of bacteria to adhere to the walls of the urinary tract. These tart berries native to North America also contain vitamin C and dietary fiber.
- **Grapefruit**—The appeal of grapefruit extends beyond the nutrients it contains, such as a significant amount of vitamin C. Grapefruit contains phytonutrients called limonoids that promote the formation of a detoxifying enzyme. Whenever possible, you should buy red or pink grapefruit rather than white; the rosy-hued grapefruit gets its pigmentation from lycopene, which is the same antioxidant found in tomatoes.
- **Grapes/Raisins**—Much has been written about resveratrol, a flavonoid in red wine that is thought to reduce the risk of heart disease, and since red wine comes from red grapes, the same hypothesis applies. In addition, grapes are an excellent source of manganese. In their dried form, raisins, they also supply the trace mineral boron, which prevents bone loss.
- **Kiwifruit**—While citrus fruits are touted for being great sources of vitamin C, no fruit can match this New Zealand native. Per gram it contains 10 percent more vitamin C than citrus fruits. Moreover, the bright green flesh of the kiwi contains powerful antioxidants, some of which are believed to protect DNA in the nucleus of cells from free radicals.

- **Mangoes**—Aromatic and juicy mangoes are a terrific source of vitamin C, and they are also high in beta-carotene, which your body converts to vitamin A. Mango is a wonderful fruit to pair with other tropical treats like pineapple and coconut, and it is equally compatible with fruits from cooler climes like strawberries.
- **Oranges**—We all know that a glass of fresh orange juice is a great way to start the day and add a boost to your immune system—in fact, studies have recently shown that drinking orange juice is actually a better way to assimilate vitamin C into the body than taking it as a nutritional supplement. One orange contains 116 percent of the vitamin C you need in a day, and it is also a good source of dietary fiber and folate. Oranges also contain a wide variety of phytonutrient compounds.
- **Papaya**—This specialty of the tropics contains an abundance of nutrients: It is a superb source of vitamin C and folate, and it contains a healthy amount of potassium and vitamins A and E. Additionally, papaya has a very high flavonoid content.
- **Pineapple**—The taste of juicy pineapple is a lovely balance of sweet and tart. No fruit is a better source of manganese in the diet, and it is also high in vitamin C. Another bonus: Pineapple contains bromelain, an enzyme that aids in digestion and reduces inflammation.
- **Plums/Prunes**—While plums are a moderate source of vitamin C, the great health benefit derived from both plums and their dried form, prunes, is their high amount of polyphenols, a very powerful antioxidant. And prunes are an excellent way to bulk up the fiber in your diet.
- **Raspberries**—Like blackberries, raspberries are a member of the rose family. They pack an antioxidant punch, plus they have a very high concentration of ellagic acid, a powerful phytonutrient. In addition, they are an excellent source of manganese, vitamin C, and dietary fiber.
- **Strawberries**—The polyphenols in strawberries are responsible for their bright red color and also give them the antioxidant power to guard against heart disease and inflammation. A superb source of vitamin C, strawberries also contain a significant amount of manganese and dietary fiber.
- **Tomatoes**—Tomatoes, along with eggplant, are actually a fruit, although we enjoy them as vegetables. Tomatoes have been much in the news recently due to the fact that their vivid red color comes from a high concentration of lycopene, a powerful antioxidant that may prevent heart disease. In addition, they are rich in both vitamin C and vitamin A.

- **Watermelon**—Tomatoes aren't the only fruit to offer you the antioxidant protection of lycopene; watermelon is another excellent source. This low-calorie fruit also contains vitamins A and B6.

Nuts and Seeds

While nuts are high in calories and contain fat, they contain "good fat" that is monounsaturated and therefore heart healthy. Nuts and seeds add a subtle flavor to smoothies, and they also serve as a thickening agent. Here are the nuts and seeds you will find in this book's smoothie recipes:

- **Almonds**—Just one-quarter cup of these delicately flavored and versatile nuts contains almost half the vitamin E and manganese you need in the course of a day, and almonds are high in heart-healthy monounsaturated fat. It is best to leave on their skins, which contain about twenty flavonoids similar to those found in green tea. Almonds are also high in protein.
- **Brazil nuts**—These huge nuts with a mild flavor and buttery texture are hands down the best vegetarian source of selenium, a trace mineral you need on a daily basis. Like all nuts, they also contain a high amount of monounsaturated fat.
- **Cashews**—Cashews have a lower fat content than most nuts, and about three-quarters of their fat is unsaturated and very high in oleic acid, the same "healthy" fat found in olive oil. These buttery and mild nuts are also an excellent source of minerals; one serving provides almost half the copper you need in a day and they are also high in magnesium and phosphorus.
- **Peanuts**—Peanuts are technically legumes, like lentils and garbanzo beans, but since we eat them like a nut, they are included on this list. Peanuts are high in manganese and other minerals, and they are a good source of resveratrol, an important antioxidant flavonoid.
- **Sesame seeds**—Both sesame seeds and tahini, the paste made from them, are loaded with necessary minerals. They are an excellent source of copper, manganese, tryptophan, calcium, magnesium, iron, and phosphorus and a good source of zinc.
- **Sunflower seeds**—I grow sunflowers in the summer to ensure a cache of organic seeds for the rest of the year. Sunflower seeds are the most nutritious snack around, and their mildly nutty flavor adds texture to smoothies. They are a superb source of vitamin E and vitamin B1, as well as many minerals, including manganese and magnesium.
- **Walnuts**—Your body cannot manufacture omega-3 fatty acids, so these essential nutrients must come from the foods we eat. Just one-quarter cup of walnuts provides more than 90 percent of the recom-

mended Daily Value of omega-3s. In addition to promoting cardio-vascular health, omega-3s are also excellent in quelling any sort of inflammation, from skin rashes to asthma to rheumatoid arthritis.

THE SUPPORTING PLAYERS

While fruits are the "stars" of your smoothies, the ingredients listed in this section rev up the drinks' nutritional value. Some, such as green tea or honey, add flavor to the smoothie while others, such as tofu, help to create a smooth texture. All of these items can be found in health food stores, and most can now be found in regular supermarkets too. Here are the "bonus" ingredients you will find in these smoothie recipes:

- **Bee pollen**—When flower seeds stick to bees' legs as they are making honey, the seeds get deposited along the sides of the hive and are harvested as bee pollen. This flavorless powder contains protein and vitamins B, C, and E and is a good source of calcium and magnesium.
- **Flaxseed oil**—Adding a salmon fillet to a smoothie might not taste very appetizing, so flaxseed oil, with its subtly nutty flavor, is the perfect alternative for incorporating omega-3 fatty acids into your diet. Instead of using flaxseed oil, you could grind flaxseeds in the blender, but I find that their hard shells add a gritty texture to the drink.
- **Green tea**—There are four polyphenols in green tea, collectively referred to as catechins, which are powerful antioxidants and have been proven effective in protecting cells throughout the body.
- **Honey**—This miraculous substance generated by bees and flowers has more sweetness than refined sugar, and it is also loaded with nutrients instead of the empty calories of granulated sugar. Honey has been used over the centuries to salve wounds, and studies have shown that it can lower cholesterol. The subtle flavor nuances of honey change depending on the particular flower the bees were working on, and in general raw honey is a better choice than processed honey because it contains far more nutrients.
- **Soy foods**—Soy in all its forms is a wonder food, and it is the only plant source of complete protein. Both soy milk and silken tofu add creaminess to smoothies without adding dairy for those who are lactose intolerant. Silken tofu is the creamiest tofu as it has had almost none of its liquid extracted. Soy foods are also good sources of manganese, iron, and selenium.
- **Whey protein powder**—Like bee pollen, whey protein powder adds nutrients but not flavor to your smoothies. Although the exact mechanisms are not fully understood, whey proteins appear to

boost production of glutathione, a fundamental part of the immune system. Whey protein powder delivers a complete protein (one that contains all the amino acids in the correct proportion) that is also high in essential amino acids.

- **Yogurt**—Acidophilus, the friendly bacteria that causes milk to coagulate and turn to yogurt, is beneficial to a healthy digestive system, and it can prevent harmful bacteria from forming. Like all dairy products, yogurt is an excellent source of calcium and also contains protein and many of the B vitamins.

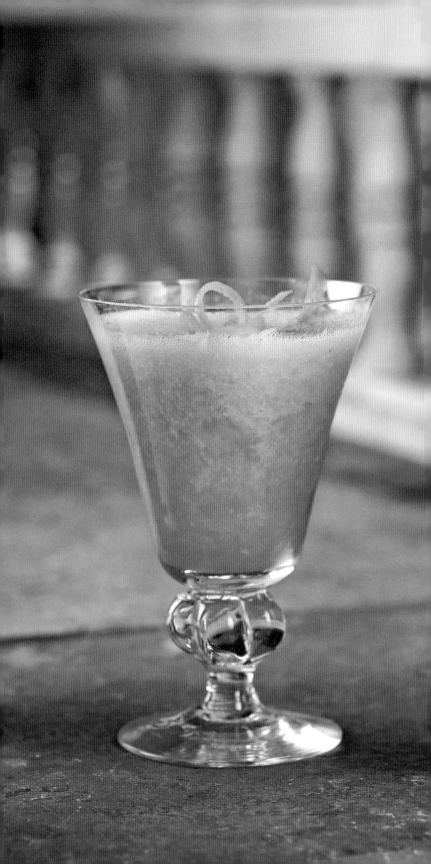

CHAPTER 3
SMOOTHIE BASICS

The good news is that these nutrient-packed drinks are incredibly easy to make; if you can push a button, you can make a smoothie. And chances are you already own a blender—the key appliance you need for making smoothies. If not, it is a small investment for the substantial benefits that drinking smoothies can bring to your health.

The blender is your secret to smoothie success because it has the power to create a thick and frosty concoction from a combination of chilled and frozen ingredients on which all smoothies are based. In this chapter you will learn about blenders, the simple logic of smoothie-making, and how to "dress up" the finished drink with super easy and healthful garnishes.

THE SMOOTHIE FAMILY TREE

Smoothies have been around since the first blender was invented in the early 1920s by Wisconsin native Stephen Poplawski. Its introduction and popularization evolved over the next decade through a maze of partner-ships, the first being between Fred Osius, one of the original principals in the Hamilton Beach company, and gadget-guru Fred Waring, better known as the singer and band leader of Fred Waring and the Pennsylvanians. They unveiled the "Miracle Mixer" in 1933, and shortly thereafter parted com-pany. Waring then improved on the concept, and introduced the Waring "Blendor" in 1939. (Interestingly, the pamphlet that accompanied the new product talked about fruit-based drinks.)

Mabel Stegner, a food writer from the now defunct *New York Herald Tribune*, wrote in 1940 about the wonders of these new blenders in making both fruit and vegetable drinks. Following World War II, these drinks became consistent with Americans' newly casual, more suburban lifestyle, in which cookouts on the patio began replacing formal meals in the dining room.

The country's developing taste for frothy fruit drinks can also be tied to the development of the Orange Julius franchise (part of Dairy Queen since 1987). The franchise got its start in California in the mid-1920s as an orange juice stand. After a few years, the stand began selling a more creamy orange juice drink, designed to be less bothersome to the stomach than the regular, acidic orange juice. By the Great Depression, there were more than one hundred outlets, and in 1964 the Orange Julius was named the official drink at the New York World's Fair.

The word "smoothie" gained public acceptance much more recently, and the first person to coin the term is anyone's guess. In the late 1950s surfboard-toting health aficionados began requesting vegetable and fruit drinks at counters in health food stores, and—like most American food trends over the past sixty years—the shops that sprouted in California eventually moved east.

By the early 1960s, when former soda jerk Stephen Kuhnau launched the Smoothie King brand, the name had already become quite popular. On the West Coast, the largest purveyor was the Juice Club, which changed its name to Jamba Juice in 1999.

CHOOSING AND USING A BLENDER OR SMOOTHIE MAKER

In many kitchens, a food processor has taken the place of a blender, and as much as I depend on my food processor, blenders really do a better job at making smoothies. The large blade and the overall shape of a food processor's work bowl do not aerate the smoothie mixture to produce a creamy, thick texture to the same degree as a blender. Additionally, food processors do not crush ice as effectively; therefore, if you plan to use a food processor to make a smoothie, you should first crush the ice into pieces no larger than a lima bean.

If you already own a blender, you are all set to make a sumptuous smoothie. If you are going to purchase a blender, however, or want to upgrade your present model, here are some criteria to keep in mind:

- Buy a machine with a heavy base to stabilize and keep it from jumping around the counter. Try lifting a number of blenders in the store, and then choose the one that feels heaviest.
- Compare brands to find one with a strong motor. A heavy-duty motor of 60 hertz or more will not only chop ice and frozen fruit with ease; it will also last far longer than machines with less power.
- Select a model with a large capacity. The beaker of a blender should never be more than two-thirds full, so one that holds forty ounces (1 1/4 L)—the most popular size for blenders made today—will easily accommodate any of the recipes in this book.
- Choose a blender with a glass beaker rather than one made from plastic. Plastic beakers scratch over time, which makes them more difficult to clean, and many plastic beakers are not dishwasher safe. Some top-of-the-line blenders are crafted completely from stainless steel—the best of both possible worlds for durability and ease of cleaning—but my personal preference is glass, which allows me to see the action in the beaker as the smoothie turns to a purée. And as accidents can happen, if you find yourself deciding between two

similar machines, buy the one whose replacement beaker is less expensive and/or easier to obtain.

- Take notice of the lid construction and make sure it consists of two pieces. This is necessary for adding frozen ingredients through the hole once your chilled ingredients are puréed. Also check that the lid fits tightly and that the smaller piece locks firmly into place.
- Choose a blender with a variety of speeds and the ability to "pulse" ingredients. While high and low speeds are universal, additional speeds are useful for breaking down your frozen ingredients into small pieces before the drink becomes a thick purée. The ability to push a quick "On" and "Off" pulsing switch is another helpful feature, both for smoothies and for general use.

If you plan to leave the blender on the kitchen counter, pick one that you find aesthetically appealing; blenders range from simple to sleek and come in a variety of colors.

Smoothie-Specific Machines

The new kid on the blender block is called a smoothie maker, and most are priced comparably to middle-to-high-end blenders. The beaker looks similar to that of a blender, but it has a spigot at the bottom so you can dispense the mixture directly from the beaker into a glass.

Convenient storage is the price you will pay for convenient serving. The bases of smoothie makers are higher than those of blenders, allowing you to position a glass beneath the spigot. The smoothie maker's higher base makes it difficult to store in many kitchen cabinets, even if you remove the beaker.

Finally, while any blender can make a smoothie, smoothie makers are not as valuable as a general cooking tool. The spigot tends to get clogged with finely chopped foods, such as nuts or breadcrumbs, and it is difficult to clean.

Safety First

As with all electrical appliances, the first precaution is to remember that a blender should be grounded and the cord should not be frayed in any way. Always unplug the blender before wiping the base clean, and never submerge the base in water; scrub it on the counter and rinse with a sponge or paper towels.

If you keep in mind that a blender has the power to crush ice and purée frozen fruit within seconds, you will understand that while it may look innocuous, a blender is a machine you should handle with care. Here are some tips on how best to use it:

- Cut all food for blending into small pieces of uniform size. An ice cube is about the largest size that can be successfully puréed.
- Never fill a blender more than two-thirds full. As the blade whirls, it will increase the volume of the liquid.

- Always keep a hand on top of the lid to ensure that it does not fly off.
- Never put your hands in the blender beaker, and make sure the blades have stopped moving before inserting a rubber spatula into the jar. Do not use metal implements inside the blender beaker.
- Turn off the blender and wait for the liquid to stop moving before removing the lid.
- An easy way to clean the blender after use is to add a few teaspoons of dishwashing liquid to the beaker and fill it half full with hot water. Blend the soapy solution for twenty seconds and rinse. If you plan to wash the beaker in the dishwasher, remove and disassemble the blade assembly from the bottom of the beaker. Wash the beaker and blade assembly components, but do not put the rubber washer in the dishwasher because the heat of the drying cycle can destroy it.

HOW TO MAKE A LUSCIOUS SMOOTHIE

To make a smoothie you need something solid to thicken the mixture, something liquid to give it a drinkable consistency, and something to bind these two categories of ingredients once they have been emulsified.

In general, a smoothie's thickness is determined by the proportion of frozen ingredients to liquid ingredients. The greater number of frozen ingredients, the thicker the smoothie will be. If you like really chilled and really thick smoothies, you should use more frozen ingredients. If you like your drinks only slightly thicker than fruit juice, then make the smoothie from only chilled ingredients (you will still achieve some thickness from the fiber in the fruit).

The higher the water content of a particular fruit, the less texture it will add to the drink. For example, slices of banana will make a smoothie far thicker than cubes of watermelon. Watermelon is more than 90 percent water, so once it is puréed, you have a lot of pink water without much texture. Another quality of fruit that dictates how much texture it will add to the smoothie is the amount of fiber it contains. Pineapple, for instance, has more fiber than peaches, so it will add more body to the drink. The fiber content is listed for each smoothie recipe, so you will be able to judge which fruits offer the most fiber.

Blending Protocol

The first step in making a smoothie is to briefly blend any liquids and other refrigerated ingredients. This initial blending creates a matrix in which it is easier to purée the frozen ingredients. The length of time required for this initial blending is determined by what ingredients are being blended. If the mixture is primarily liquid, or a soft solid like yogurt or silken tofu, then twenty seconds is sufficient. However, if your chilled ingredients include such fibrous foods as strawberries or apples, forty-five seconds is the rec- ommended time. But let your eye be the judge; you want these ingredients to be totally puréed before adding frozen ingredients to the beaker.

If you decide to use ingredients in a different form than how they are listed in the recipe, you should reverse the order in which they are added. For example, if you choose to add frozen blueberries rather than chilled, add them at the end of the recipe rather than at the beginning. Just remem- ber the rule that frozen ingredients go last.

If you wish to modify a smoothie recipe, feel free to do so—but limit your changes to the same category of ingredient. For example, if you wish to substitute soy milk for cow's milk or frozen tofu for ice cream, that is an appropriate and easy substitution because they are the same category of ingredient. However, if you substitute soy milk for one of the fruits in the recipe, your drink will not have the proper consistency.

In addition to having something liquid and something frozen, most smoothies also contain an ingredient or two that provides a creamy texture—these are referred to as binders. This might be a dairy product such as yogurt or frozen yogurt, a creamy product such as silken tofu, or any number of nutritional supplements. Whey protein powder and bee pollen lend a very creamy texture to smoothies.

Certain medical conditions, such as diverticulitis, can be aggravated by the seeds in fruits such as strawberries. If you would prefer to strain your smoothie, do so before adding the frozen ingredients.

Dressing Up a Smoothie

Part of the fun of serving smoothies is that health never tasted quite so delicious, and if time permits, you might consider embellishing the glass with a garnish. After all, we eat with our eyes before the first sip reaches our lips. It is easy to dress up smoothies because their thick texture means you can float almost anything on their surface. And besides adding color and decoration, the garnish lends texture to the eating experience.

Here are several garnish ideas that are simple to create:

- **Fruit kebabs**—Reserve some of the fruit used in the smoothie and thread bite-sized pieces onto a toothpick or other decorative spear. For a fancier look, use a combination of different fruits.
- **Strawberry fans**—Reserve large strawberries for the garnish, but do not remove their green caps after rinsing. Use a sharp paring knife to make five or six slices through the berry, beginning at the cap. Transfer the strawberry to a plate, and gently spread the slices apart to form a fan.
- **Fruit spears**—Fruits such as peaches, melons, mango, papaya, and pineapple are large and sturdy enough to use without toothpicks. Cut the fruit into thin slices and either poise it on the rim of the glass or lay it on top of the smoothie.

- **Cookies**—Any crisp cookie, especially a rolled pirouette, looks pretty peeking out of the top of a smoothie, and the cookie serves as an inducement for children to finish their drink.
- **Chocolate shavings**—Use the large holes of a box grater to grate a chocolate bar. Sprinkle the shavings over the top of the smoothie.
- **Chocolate-dipped fruit**—This garnish involves a bit of effort, but it adds both a nutritious fruit and the indulgence of chocolate to your smoothie. Using either white or dark chocolate, chop the chocolate finely, and melt it either in a double boiler over simmering water or in the microwave. (If you use a microwave, set on medium power for thirty-second intervals, stirring the chocolate as it melts.) The fruits that work best for dipping are those that are fairly dry, such as strawberries (rinsed and patted dry on paper towels), or large dried fruit, such as dried apricots or dried pineapple. Dip the fruit in the melted chocolate, and lay it on a sheet of plastic wrap or waxed paper until the chocolate has set.
- **Sprinkling of spices**—Cinnamon and nutmeg provide flavor and an aromatic note as a garnish, and their dark color adds visual interest.
- **Non-edible garnishes**—Decorations such as pineapple leaves or a knot made from a thin slice of orange peel can add aesthetic appeal and contrasting color to a smoothie. And don't forget about those little paper umbrellas used in tropical drinks. Kids—and even adults—adore them!

Serving Smoothies for Dessert

While smoothies can be served with some simple cookies for a delicious dessert, you can also go one step further and turn your smoothie into your own homemade frozen treat, similar in texture and flavor to ice cream or frozen yogurt. And you don't need an expensive machine to accomplish this task (although it can be done in an ice cream maker if you own one).

In either case, make the smoothie according to the recipe directions. If using an ice cream machine, follow the manufacturer's instructions after preparing the smoothie. If not using an ice cream machine, pour the smoothie mixture into a 9x13-inch (23x33-cm) pan, and place it in the freezer. When it has partially frozen—the consistency will be similar to that of a snow cone—scrape the mixture into a mixing bowl and beat it well with an electric mixer. Repeat this entire process two more times, then scrape the mixture into a storage container and freeze until solid. Enjoy!

CHAPTER 4
RECIPES FOR SUPER SMOOTHIES

Now that you know why you should eat more fresh fruits, nuts, seeds, and other natural ingredients to boost your immune system, and you know which foods offer which nutrients, it's time to start enjoying good health by drinking delicious smoothies!

In this chapter you'll find one hundred drinks you can make within a matter of minutes. Each recipe is annotated with both a basic nutritional analysis and an analysis of key nutrients directly tied to the health of your immune system.

The recipes are arranged according to their dominant ingredient, so if you have ripe bananas on hand, for example, you will find all the recipes that feature them listed together. Feel free to consult the index, too; while pineapple might be the centerpiece in one recipe, it may have a secondary role to mango or papaya in another, so the index will be useful in directing you to every option for a particular food.

FRESH FROM THE FREEZER

In each recipe, one or more frozen ingredients is utilized to create the drink's characteristically thick texture. This ingredient can be as simple as ice cubes made from green tea, fruit juice, or water, but most often it is fruit that has been frozen in advance.

Freezing fruit is both easy and economical; you can purchase fruit when it is at its peak ripeness and then freeze it for up to three months. Keep in mind that the pieces should be no larger than an ice cube. This is not a problem with blueberries, raspberries, or most strawberries, of course, but fruits such as peaches and pineapple will require slicing and dicing.

Rinse all fruits and peel them if necessary. For fruits such as peaches or apricots, peeling is an optional step, but it is required for cantaloupe, pineapple, and kiwi. Then arrange the pieces on a cookie sheet covered with a sheet of plastic wrap. Once they are frozen solid, transfer the pieces to a heavy resealable plastic bag and store in the freezer. (If you are in a hurry to make your smoothie, cut the fruit into very small pieces. These should freeze within thirty minutes.) If you buy packages of frozen fruit in the supermarket, select fruit that is dry-packed in bags rather than packed in syrup. Happy sipping!

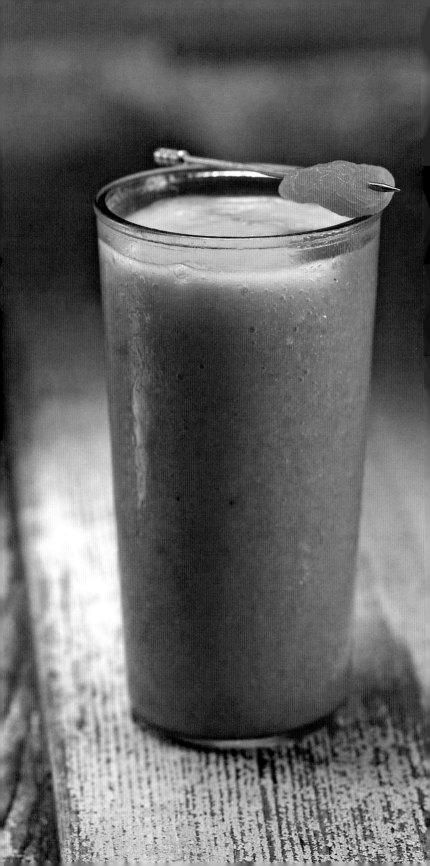

B-BOOSTING
BANANA APRICOT SMOOTHIE

You cannot find a fruit with as much essential vitamin B6—which helps maintain the health of your organs—as bananas. They are also rich in potassium, an important mineral that balances the electrolytes in your body, especially after exercise. A banana's mild flavor and creamy texture makes it a natural to match with perky apricots, a good source of vitamin A and the antioxidant lycopene.

> 1 1/2 cups (355 ml) chilled apricot nectar
> 3 fresh apricots, seeded and diced
> 2 ounces (55 g) dried apricots, diced
> 1/4 cup (32 g) whey protein powder
> 2 tablespoons (30 g) bee pollen
> 2 cups (300 g) banana slices, frozen
> 4 dried apricots for garnish (optional)

■ Combine apricot nectar, fresh apricots, dried apricots, whey protein powder, and bee pollen in a blender or smoothie maker. Blend on high speed for 45 seconds or until mixture is puréed and smooth. Add banana slices, and blend on high speed again until mixture is smooth. Serve immediately, garnished with dried apricots, if desired.

■ **YIELD:** Four 1-cup (235-ml) servings

■ **NUTRITIONAL ANALYSIS:** Each 1-cup serving provides 227 calories; 1 g total fat; 0.5 g saturated fat; 4 g protein; 55 g carbohydrate; 5 g dietary fiber; 0 mg cholesterol.

■ **TIP:** Even bright green bananas will ripen to perfection in three days if you place them in a brown paper bag, together with a few apples, at room temperature. Apples release a gas that causes bananas to ripen faster.

SUPERCHARGE NUTRIENTS:	% DAILY VALUE*
Vitamin A	3025.7 IU (61%)
Vitamin B6	0.7 mg (37%)
Vitamin C	48 mg (80%)
Vitamin E	.1.2 mg (6%)
Magnesium	50.5 mg (13%)
Manganese	0.3 mg (13%)
Selenium	1.9 mcg (3%)
Zinc	0.9 mg (13%)

* Percent Daily Values are based on a 2,000 calorie diet. Your daily values may be higher or lower depending on your caloric needs.

CULLING THE COPPER
BANANA SESAME SMOOTHIE

Copper is the mineral linked most often with relieving the pain of rheumatoid arthritis, a prevalent autoimmune disease, and sesame seeds— the basis for tahini—are among the best sources of this trace mineral. Their flavor is subtle and blends nicely with that of potassium-rich bananas.

1 cup (235 ml) plain soy milk
1/2 cup (120 ml) silken tofu
1/2 cup (120 g) tahini
1/4 cup (30 g) sesame seeds
1/4 cup (85 g) honey
2 tablespoons (30 g) bee pollen
1/2 teaspoon (2.5 ml) pure vanilla extract
2 cups (300 g) banana slices, frozen
2 tablespoons (15 g) toasted sesame seeds for garnish (optional)

■ Combine soy milk, tofu, tahini, sesame seeds, honey, bee pollen, and vanilla extract in a blender or smoothie maker. Blend on high speed for 20 seconds or until mixture is puréed and smooth. Add banana slices, and blend on high speed again until mixture is smooth. Serve immediately, garnished with sesame seeds, if desired.

■ **YIELD:** Four 1-cup (235-ml) servings

■ **NUTRITIONAL ANALYSIS:** Each 1-cup serving provides 298 calories; 9 g total fat; 1.5 g saturated fat; 6 g protein; 52 g carbohydrate; 4 g dietary fiber; 0 mg cholesterol.

■ **TIP:** Rather than sweetening foods with refined sugar—and getting nothing but empty calories—look to your honey jar. Honey is an antioxidant and contains antimicrobial properties. It has also been shown to be an effective, inexpensive, and readily available energy source for endurance athletes in place of commercial gel packs.

SUPERCHARGE NUTRIENTS:	% DAILY VALUE*
Vitamin A	224.3 IU (4%)
Vitamin B6	0.7 mg (36%)
Vitamin C	10.6 mg (18%)
Vitamin E	0.7 mg (4%)
Magnesium	82.9 mg (21%)
Manganese	0.4 mg (20%)
Selenium	3.2 mcg (5%)
Zinc	1.5 mg (10%)

* Percent Daily Values are based on a 2,000 calorie diet. Your daily values may be higher or lower depending on your caloric needs.

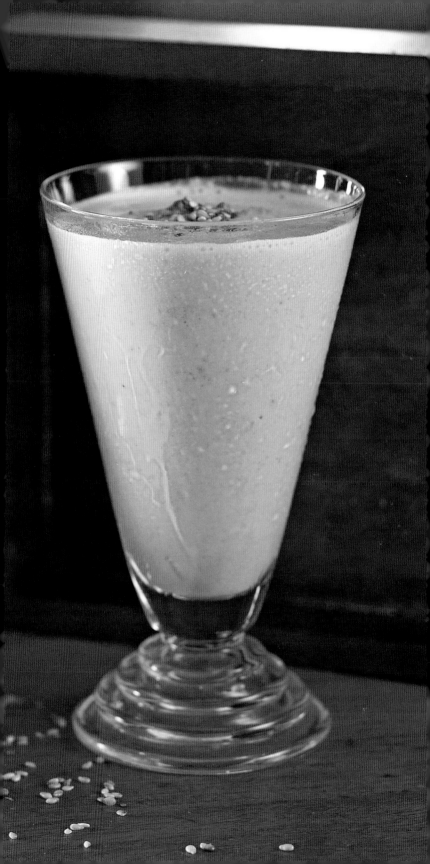

AMAZING OMEGA
BANANA MAPLE WALNUT SMOOTHIE

Omega-3 fatty acids are vital to a strong immune system because they help prevent disease, and walnuts are an excellent source of this nutrient, and walnuts also contain minerals such as manganese and copper.

1 cup (150 g) shelled walnuts
3/4 cup (175 ml) vanilla soy milk
1/2 cup (120 ml) silken tofu
1/3 cup (80 ml) pure maple syrup
1/2 cup (145 g) shelled sunflower seeds
2 tablespoons (30 g) bee pollen
1/2 teaspoon (1.2 g) ground cinnamon
2 cups (300 g) banana slices, frozen
1/2 cup (70 g) vanilla frozen yogurt
Sprinkle of ground cinnamon for garnish (optional)

■ Preheat the oven to 350°F (180°C, or gas mark 4). Place walnuts on a baking sheet, and bake for 5 to 7 minutes or until lightly browned. Remove nuts from the oven, and allow to cool completely.

■ Combine walnuts, soy milk, tofu, maple syrup, sunflower seeds, bee pollen, and cinnamon in a blender or smoothie maker. Blend on high speed for 45 seconds or until mixture is puréed and smooth. Add banana slices and frozen yogurt, and blend on high speed again until mixture is smooth. Serve immediately, garnished with a sprinkle of cinnamon, if desired.

■ **YIELD:** Four 1-cup (235-ml) servings

■ **NUTRITIONAL ANALYSIS:** Each 1-cup serving provides 486 calories; 23 g total fat; 3 g saturated fat; 14 g protein; 62 g carbohydrate; 6 g dietary fiber; 2.5 mg cholesterol.

■ **TIP:** Some people think that the skins of walnuts give foods a bitter taste. If you are one of these people, here is an easy way to remove the skins: while the nuts are still hot place them in a clean cloth towel and rub them around. The skins will slide right off.

SUPERCHARGE NUTRIENTS:	% DAILY VALUE*
Vitamin A	135.3 IU (3%)
Vitamin B6	0.7 mg (37%)
Vitamin C	14.3 mg (24%)
Vitamin E	10.3 mg (52%)
Magnesium	115.4 mg (29%)
Manganese	2.1 mg (104%)
Selenium	17.9 mcg (26%)
Zinc	2.6mg (17%)

* Percent Daily Values are based on a 2,000 calorie diet. Your daily values may be higher or lower depending on your caloric needs.

FAB FOR FIBER
RASPBERRY BANANA SMOOTHIE

Your immune system does not exist in a vacuum; it is one of the systems that your body needs to keep in working order at all times. The dietary fiber in both raspberries and bananas is important to keep your gastrointestinal system working well. The nutrients in these two fruits boost your immune system too.

> 1 container (8 ounces or 225 g) raspberry low-fat yogurt
> 1/2 cup (120 ml) silken tofu
> 1/4 cup (80 g) fruit-only raspberry preserves
> 1 cup (150 g) sliced banana
> 1/4 cup (32 g) whey protein powder
> 2 tablespoons (30 g) bee pollen
> 1 1/2 cups (190 g) raspberries, frozen
> 1/2 cup (70 g) vanilla frozen yogurt
> 12 raspberries threaded onto 4 bamboo skewers for garnish (optional)

■ Combine yogurt, tofu, raspberry preserves, banana, whey protein powder, and bee pollen in a blender or smoothie maker. Blend on high speed for 45 seconds or until mixture is puréed and smooth. Add raspberries and frozen yogurt, and blend on high speed again until mixture is smooth. Serve immediately, garnished with raspberries, if desired.

■ **YIELD:** Four 1-cup (235-ml) servings

■ **NUTRITIONAL ANALYSIS:** Each 1-cup serving provides 279 calories; 3 g total fat; 2 g saturated fat; 14 g protein; 51 g carbohydrate; 5 g dietary fiber; 24 mg cholesterol.

■ **TIP:** Keep in mind that smoothies can be made in different ways and achieve the same results. In this recipe, for example, if you had bananas already frozen, then you could add the raspberries chilled rather than frozen. What is important is that the frozen ingredient is added after those that are blended chilled.

SUPERCHARGE NUTRIENTS:	% DAILY VALUE*
Vitamin A	195.1 IU (4%)
Vitamin B6	0.3 mg (15%)
Vitamin C	22.9 mg (38%)
Vitamin E	1.0 mg (5%)
Magnesium	46.3 mg (12%)
Manganese	0.5 mg (25%)
Selenium	2.7 mcg (4%)
Zinc:	1.2 mg (8%)

* Percent Daily Values are based on a 2,000 calorie diet. Your daily values may be higher or lower depending on your caloric needs.

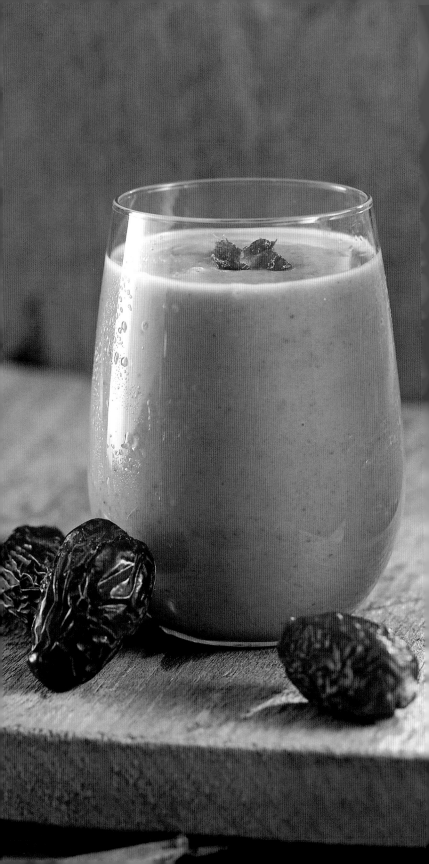

BETTER FOR B6
BANANA DATE SMOOTHIE

Your immune system needs vitamin B6 to keep the lymphoid organs healthy and producing white blood cells, and bananas are high in this water-soluble vitamin. In addition, dates contain a fair amount of iron, and their succulent flavor is the perfect foil for the subtle banana.

- 1 container (8 ounces or 225 g) banana low-fat yogurt
- 1/2 cup (120 ml) silken tofu
- 2 cups (300 g) sliced banana
- 1 cup (175 g) firmly packed pitted dried dates, diced
- 2 tablespoons (30 ml) flaxseed oil
- 2 tablespoons (30 g) bee pollen
- 1/2 cup (70 g) vanilla frozen yogurt
- 2 tablespoons (20 g) finely chopped pitted dried dates for garnish (optional)

■ Combine yogurt, tofu, bananas, dates, flaxseed oil, and bee pollen in a blender or smoothie maker. Blend on high speed for 45 seconds or until mixture is puréed and smooth. Add frozen yogurt, and blend on high speed again until mixture is smooth. Serve immediately, garnished with chopped dates, if desired.

■ **YIELD:** Four 1-cup (235-ml) servings

■ **NUTRITIONAL ANALYSIS:** Each 1-cup serving provides 293 calories; 8.5 g total fat; 2 g saturated fat; 6 g protein; 52 g carbohydrate; 4 g dietary fiber; 6 mg cholesterol.

■ **TIP:** Silken tofu has almost none of its water extracted, which is why it has the same liquid-like texture as yogurt. If you are using soft tofu in its place, add a few tablespoons of water to the recipe to achieve the proper texture.

SUPERCHARGE NUTRIENTS:	% DAILY VALUE*
Vitamin A	47.2 IU (1%)
Vitamin B6	0.2 mg (8%)
Vitamin C	4.6 mg (8%)
Vitamin E	1.8 mg (9%)
Magnesium	31.4 mg (8%)
Manganese	0.2 mg (10%)
Selenium	2.5 mcg (4%)
Zinc	0.9 mg (6%)

Percent Daily Values are based on a 2,000 calorie diet. Your daily values may be higher or lower depending on your caloric needs.

FOLATE-FILLED
TROPICAL BANANA SMOOTHIE

Folate, which is important to maintaining your red blood cell production, is easy to find in legumes like lentils, but it's far more difficult to get a sufficient quantity from fruit. Papaya is one of the exceptions. It has a sweet flavor, a ton of vitamin C, and when joined with creamy banana and flavorful coconut, it makes a great smoothie.

- 3/4 cup (175 ml) chilled papaya nectar
- 1/2 cup (120 ml) chilled light coconut milk
- 1/2 cup (120 ml) silken tofu
- 1 cup (175 g) diced papaya
- 1/2 cup (40 g) fresh shredded coconut
- 2 tablespoons (30 g) bee pollen
- 1 1/2 cups (225 g) banana slices, frozen
- 8 mango cubes for garnish (optional)

■ Combine papaya nectar, coconut milk, tofu, papaya, coconut, and bee pollen in a blender or smoothie maker. Blend on high speed for 45 seconds or until mixture is puréed and smooth. Add banana slices, and blend on high speed again until mixture is smooth. Serve immediately, garnished with mango spears, if desired.

■ **YIELD:** Four 1-cup (235-ml) servings

■ **NUTRITIONAL ANALYSIS:** Each 1-cup serving provides 248 calories; 10 g total fat; 9 g saturated fat; 4 g protein; 39 g carbohydrate; 5 g dietary fiber; 0 mg cholesterol.

■ **TIP:** Coconut milk is very high in fat, much of it saturated fat. Light coconut milk, however, contains the same nutrients, such as vitamin C and calcium, but is far lower in fat. It is therefore always the better choice.

SUPERCHARGE NUTRIENTS:	% DAILY VALUE*
Vitamin A	826.4 IU (17%)
Vitamin B6	0.6 mg (28%)
Vitamin C	35.2 mg (59%)
Vitamin E	1.4 mg (7%)
Magnesium	48.6 mg (12%)
Manganese	0.6 mg (30%)
Selenium	4.9 mcg (7%)
Zinc	1.0 mg (7%)

Percent Daily Values are based on a 2,000 calorie diet. Your daily values may be higher or lower depending on your caloric needs.

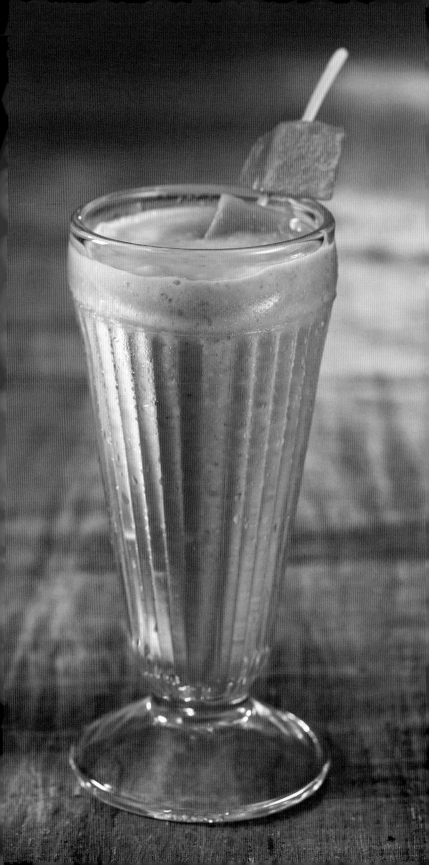

PUMP THAT POTASSIUM
BANANA ORANGE SMOOTHIE

Potassium is a mineral that your body needs to keep electrolytes in balance as well as to boost your immune system. Bananas are an excellent source of this key nutrient. Along with oranges, they are a good source of dietary fiber too, which is why this smoothie has such a rich and thick texture when you drink it.

>   2 navel oranges
>   1 container (8 ounces or 225 g) plain nonfat yogurt
>   1/2 cup (120 ml) freshly squeezed orange juice
>   1/4 cup (80 g) fruit-only orange marmalade
>   1/4 cup (32 g) whey protein powder
>   2 tablespoons (30 g) bee pollen
>   1/2 teaspoon (1.2 g) ground cinnamon
>   2 cups (300 g) banana slices, frozen
>   4 orange segments for garnish (optional)

■ Peel oranges, then slice off white pith. Cut around sides of sections to release segments from remaining pith. Cut into 1/2-inch (1-cm) dice.

■ Combine oranges, yogurt, orange juice, orange marmalade, whey protein powder, bee pollen, and cinnamon in a blender or smoothie maker. Blend on high speed for 45 seconds or until mixture is puréed and smooth. Add banana slices, and blend on high speed again until mixture is smooth. Serve immediately, garnished with orange segments, if desired.

■ **YIELD:** Four 1-cup (235-ml) servings

■ **NUTRITIONAL ANALYSIS:** Each 1-cup serving provides 280 calories; 1 g total fat; 1 g saturated fat; 13.5 g protein; 58 g carbohydrate; 4 g dietary fiber; 19.5 mg cholesterol.

■ **TIP:** It is now more common to see baby bananas on the market, as well as plantains, which are a first cousin. When ripe, both of these fruits have a sweeter flavor than the common Cavendish banana, and can be substituted in recipes.

SUPERCHARGE NUTRIENTS:	% DAILY VALUE*
Vitamin A	322.2 IU (6%)
Vitamin B6	0.5 mg (27%)
Vitamin C	65.6 mg (109%)
Vitamin E	1.1 mg (5%)
Magnesium	57.4 mg (14%)
Manganese	0.4 mg (19%)
Selenium	3.7 mcg (5%)
Zinc	1.1 mg (7%)

* Percent Daily Values are based on a 2,000 calorie diet. Your daily values may be higher or lower depending on your caloric needs.

BUILDING BLOCK
BANANA MANGO CASHEW SMOOTHIE

Like sesame and sunflower seeds, sweet and buttery cashew nuts are an excellent source of copper, a trace mineral your immune system needs to create a number of enzymes. They also add a richness to this smoothie made with aromatic mangos, which are high in vitamin C, and potassium-rich bananas.

- 1/2 cup (75 g) raw cashew nuts
- 1 container (8 ounces or 225 g) banana low-fat yogurt
- 1/2 cup (120 ml) silken tofu
- 2 cups (350 g) diced mango
- 1/4 cup (32 g) whey protein powder
- 2 tablespoons (30 ml) flaxseed oil
- 1/4 teaspoon (1.2 ml) rum extract
- 1 1/2 cups (300 g) banana slices, frozen
- 4 mango spears for garnish (optional)

▓ Preheat the oven to 350°F (180°C, or gas mark 4). Place cashews on a baking sheet, and bake for 5 to 7 minutes or until lightly browned. Remove nuts from the oven, and allow to cool completely.

▓ Combine cashews, yogurt, tofu, mango, whey protein powder, flaxseed oil, and rum extract in a blender or smoothie maker. Blend on high speed for 45 seconds or until mixture is puréed and smooth. Add banana slices, and blend on high speed again until mixture is smooth. Serve immediately, garnished with mango spears, if desired.

▓ **YIELD:** Four 1-cup (235-ml) servings

▓ **NUTRITIONAL ANALYSIS:** Each 1-cup serving provides 367 calories; 16 g total fat; 3 g saturated fat; 16 g protein; 44 g carbohydrate; 4 g dietary fiber; 20 mg cholesterol.

▓ **TIP:** While nuts can keep very well if frozen, if you are buying a small quantity the best place to look is the bulk bins at health food stores, where you can purchase only the quantity you need.

SUPERCHARGE NUTRIENTS:	% DAILY VALUE*
Vitamin A	3406.6 IU (68%)
Vitamin B6	0.5 mg (25 %)
Vitamin C	40.9 mg (68%)
Vitamin E	2.6 mg (13%)
Magnesium	96.0 mg (24%)
Manganese	0.3 mg (15%)
Selenium	3.2 mcg (5%)
Zinc	1.5 mg (10%)

* Percent Daily Values are based on a 2,000 calorie diet. Your daily values may be higher or lower depending on your caloric needs.

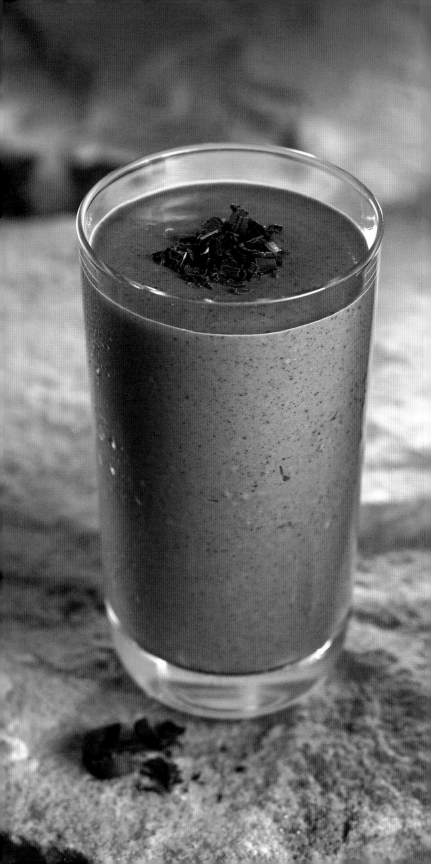

CHOLESTEROL LOWERING MEXICAN CHOCOLATE BANANA SMOOTHIE

Mexicans were the first to appreciate the wonders of hot chocolate, and their version is made with almonds and cinnamon. In addition to supplying a high content of vitamin E, which protects cell membranes against free radicals, and manganese, which helps your body metabolize fatty acids, almonds serve to prevent a rise in blood sugar after eating.

1 cup (235 ml) chocolate soy milk
1/2 cup (120 ml) silken tofu
1 cup (150 g) shelled almonds, not skinned
1/2 cup (50 g) chopped dark chocolate
2 tablespoons (30 ml) flaxseed oil
1/2 teaspoon (1.2 g) ground cinnamon
2 cups (300 g) banana slices, frozen
2 tablespoons (12.5 g) grated chocolate for garnish (optional)

▨ Combine soy milk, tofu, almonds, chocolate, flaxseed oil, and cinnamon in a blender or smoothie maker. Blend on high speed for 45 seconds or until mixture is puréed and smooth. Add banana slices, and blend on high speed again until mixture is smooth. Serve immediately, garnished with grated chocolate, if desired.

▨ **YIELD:** Four 1-cup (235-ml) servings

▨ **NUTRITIONAL ANALYSIS:** Each 1-cup serving provides 487 calories; 31 g total fat; 5 g saturated fat; 12 g protein; 50 g carbohydrate; 7 g dietary fiber; 1 mg cholesterol.

▨ **TIP:** An easy way to grate chocolate is to use the large holes on a box grater. Always remember to hold the chocolate with a paper towel: It will protect your fingers and keep their heat from melting the chocolate.

SUPERCHARGE NUTRIENTS:	% DAILY VALUE*
Vitamin A	107.9 IU (2%)
Vitamin B6	0.8 mg (39%)
Vitamin C	10.5 mg (17%)
Vitamin E	10.5 mg (52%)
Magnesium	164.0 mg (41%)
Manganese	1.3 mg (65%)
Selenium	5.6 mcg (8%)
Zinc	2.0 mg (13%)

* Percent Daily Values are based on a 2,000 calorie diet. Your daily values may be higher or lower depending on your caloric needs.

GUILT-FREE
BANANA CHOCOLATE SMOOTHIE

Great news for chocoholics: Dark chocolate contains the same heart-healthy flavonoids as red wine, so it, too, can help lower our cholesterol. In fact, one Dutch study showed that chocolate contains four times the amount of catechins as tea! This smoothie contains not one but *two* forms of chocolate and is thickened by rich, creamy banana.

1 1/2 cups (355 ml) chocolate soy milk
3 ounces (85 g) chopped dark chocolate
3 tablespoons (45 g) cocoa powder, preferably Dutch-processed
2 tablespoons (30 g) bee pollen
2 tablespoons (30 ml) flaxseed oil
2 cups (300 g) sliced banana
1 cup (140 g) chocolate frozen yogurt
2 tablespoons (15 g) shaved chocolate for garnish (optional)

▨ Combine soy milk, chopped chocolate, cocoa powder, bee pollen, flaxseed oil, and banana in a blender or smoothie maker. Blend on high speed for 45 seconds or until mixture is puréed and smooth. Add frozen yogurt, and blend on high speed again until mixture is smooth. Serve immediately, garnished with chocolate shavings, if desired.

▨ **YIELD:** Four 1-cup (235-ml) servings

▨ **NUTRITIONAL ANALYSIS:** Each 1-cup serving provides 470 calories; 19 g total fat; 6 g saturated fat; 11 g protein; 71 g carbohydrate; 4 g dietary fiber; 5 mg cholesterol.

▨ **TIP:** Rather than having to rely on a measuring cup for ice cream or frozen yogurt, measure the capacity of your ice cream scoop. From that point on, you can use the scoop for measuring purposes and you will have one less utensil to wash.

SUPERCHARGE NUTRIENTS:	% DAILY VALUE*
Vitamin A	220.6 IU (4%)
Vitamin B6	0.8 mg (40%)
Vitamin C	14.8 mg (25%)
Vitamin E	2.4 mg (12%)
Magnesium	106.0 mg (27%)
Manganese	0.4 mg (18%)
Selenium	.13 mcg (2%)
Zinc	1.7 mg (12%)

* Percent Daily Values are based on a 2,000 calorie diet. Your daily values may be higher or lower depending on your caloric needs.

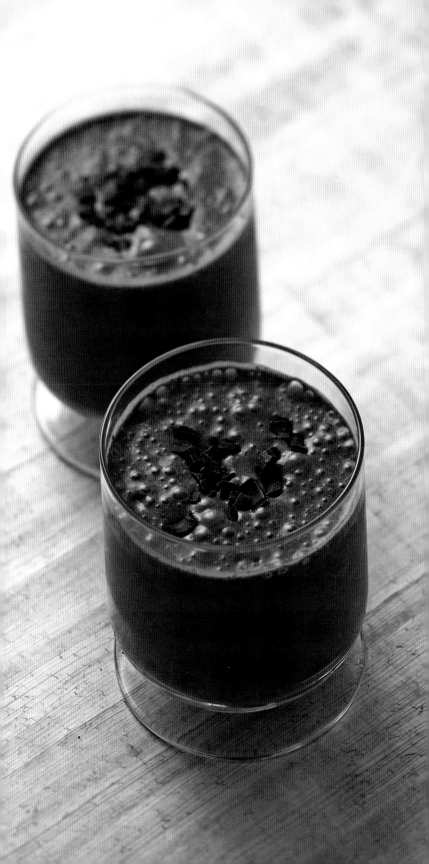

LUSCIOUS LEGUME
CHOCOLATE PEANUT BANANA SMOOTHIE

Resveratrol is a powerful antioxidant, and it is best known as a nutrient found in red grapes and red wine. But peanuts, a member of the legume family, are also a good source of resveratrol, and when they are blended with potassium-rich bananas, you are rewarded with a delicious smoothie high in many vital trace minerals.

> 1 cup (235 ml) chocolate soy milk
> 1/2 cup (120 ml) silken tofu
> 1/2 cup (130 g) natural peanut butter
> 1/2 cup (72 g) shelled peanuts
> 1/2 cup (50 g) chopped dark chocolate
> 1/4 cup (32 g) whey protein powder
> 2 tablespoons (30 ml) flaxseed oil
> 2 tablespoons (40 g) honey
> 2 tablespoons (30 g) bee pollen
> 1 1/2 cups (225 g) banana slices, frozen
> 2 tablespoons chopped peanuts for garnish (optional)

■ Combine soy milk, tofu, peanut butter, peanuts, chocolate, whey protein powder, flaxseed oil, honey, and bee pollen in a blender or smoothie maker. Blend on high speed for 45 seconds or until mixture is puréed and smooth. Add banana slices, and blend on high speed again until mixture is smooth. Serve immediately, garnished with chopped peanuts, if desired.

■ **YIELD:** Four 1-cup (235-ml) servings

■ **NUTRITIONAL ANALYSIS:** Each 1-cup serving provides 662 calories; 38 g total fat; 8 g saturated fat; 27 g protein; 56 g carbohydrate; 6 g dietary fiber; 20 mg cholesterol.

■ **TIP:** Natural peanut butter is carried in most supermarkets as well as health food markets. It usually needs to be stirred well because the oil rises to the top. If you are using commercial peanut butter, omit the honey to compensate for the included sugar.

SUPERCHARGE NUTRIENTS:	% DAILY VALUE*
Vitamin A	102.5 IU (2%)
Vitamin B6	0.6 mg (30%)
Vitamin C	11.6 mg (19%)
Vitamin E	3.3 mg (16%)
Magnesium	143.0 mg (36%)
Manganese	0.6 mg (29%)
Selenium	1.5 mcg (2%)
Zinc	1.5 mg (10%)

* Percent Daily Values are based on a 2,000 calorie diet. Your daily values may be higher or lower depending on your caloric needs.

FANCY PHYTONUTRIENT BANANA CHOCOLATE RASPBERRY SMOOTHIE

The great news for chocolate lovers is that dark chocolate actually contains nutrients; it is not just empty calories. When the phytonutrients in dark chocolate combine with the ellagic acid in raspberries and the healthful content of bananas, the result is a treat that is truly good for you!

1 container (8 ounces or 225 g) raspberry low-fat yogurt
1/4 cup (80 g) fruit-only raspberry preserves
3 ounces (85 g) chopped dark chocolate
1 1/2 cups (225 g) sliced banana
3 tablespoons (45 g) cocoa powder, preferably Dutch-processed
2 tablespoons (30 g) bee pollen
2 tablespoons (30 ml) flaxseed oil
1 cup (125 g) raspberries, frozen
1/2 cup (70 g) chocolate frozen yogurt
Sprinkle of cocoa powder for garnish (optional)

▓ Combine yogurt, raspberry preserves, chocolate, banana, cocoa powder, bee pollen, and flaxseed oil in a blender or smoothie maker. Blend on high speed for 45 seconds or until mixture is puréed and smooth. Add raspberries and frozen yogurt, and blend on high speed again until mixture is smooth. Serve immediately, garnished with a sprinkling of cocoa, if desired.

▓ **YIELD:** Four 1-cup (235-ml) servings

▓ **NUTRITIONAL ANALYSIS:** Each 1-cup serving provides 481 calories; 18.5 g total fat; 6 g saturated fat; 9 g protein; 73 g carbohydrate; 6 g dietary fiber; 10.1 mg cholesterol.

▓ **TIP:** Cocoa powder is made when chocolate liquor is pressed to remove at least three-quarters of its cocoa butter, but it is done in two ways. Dutch-processed cocoa is treated with an alkali to neutralize its acids, and the resulting powder has a delicate flavor that makes it preferable for smoothies because there is no cooking to mellow the cocoa.

SUPERCHARGE NUTRIENTS:	% DAILY VALUE*
Vitamin A	287.8 IU (6%)
Vitamin B6	0.4 mg (22%)
Vitamin C	23.2 mg (39%)
Vitamin E	2.2 mg (11%)
Magnesium	70.4 mg (18%)
Manganese	0.5 mg (24%)
Selenium	3.3 mcg (5%)
Zinc	1.5 mg (10%)

* Percent Daily Values are based on a 2,000 calorie diet. Your daily values may be higher or lower depending on your caloric needs.

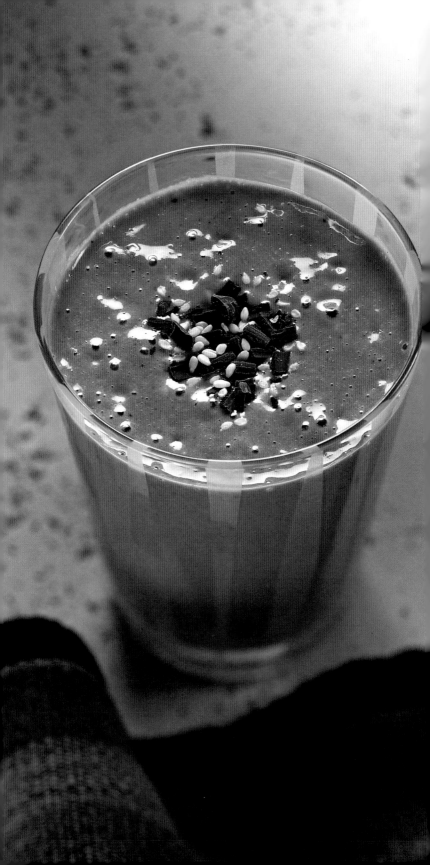

CALMING TRYPTOPHAN
SESAME CHOCOLATE BANANA SMOOTHIE

Tryptophan is among the essential amino acids that your body cannot synthesize and must therefore get from your diet. The precursor of serotonin, tryptophan also has a calming effect that can lead to relaxation and sleep. Sesame seeds and tofu are good sources of tryptophan and are packed with immune-boosting nutrients, so they balance the small amount of caffeine in the chocolate in this luscious smoothie.

   1 cup (235 ml) chocolate soy milk
   1/2 cup (120 ml) silken tofu
   1/3 cup (80 g) tahini
   1/4 cup (32 g) whey protein powder
   1/4 cup (30 g) sesame seeds
   2 tablespoons (28 ml) chocolate syrup
   1/4 teaspoon (1 ml) pure vanilla extract
   2 cups (300 g) banana slices, frozen
   2 tablespoons (15 g) toasted sesame seeds and/or chocolate shavings
      for garnish (optional)

▓ Combine soy milk, tofu, tahini, whey protein powder, sesame seeds, chocolate syrup, and vanilla extract in a blender or smoothie maker. Blend on high speed for 45 seconds or until mixture is puréed and smooth. Add banana slices, and blend on high speed again until mixture is smooth. Serve immediately, garnished with sesame seeds, if desired.

▓ **YIELD:** Four 1-cup (235-ml) servings

▓ **NUTRITIONAL ANALYSIS:** Each 1-cup serving provides 376 calories; 16 g total fat; 3 g saturated fat; 15 g protein; 48 g carbohydrate; 4 g dietary fiber; 18 mg cholesterol.

▓ **TIP:** Sesame seeds add texture to the finished drink, but if you do not have them on hand or prefer a smoother smoothie, you can omit the sesame seeds and increase the amount of tahini to one-half cup.

SUPERCHARGE NUTRIENTS:	% DAILY VALUE*
Vitamin A	122.0 IU (2%)
Vitamin B6	0.8 mg (39%)
Vitamin C	11.3 mg (19%)
Vitamin E	0.6 mg (3%)
Magnesium	106.4 mg (27%)
Manganese	0.3 mg (14%)
Selenium	3.5 mcg (5%)
Zinc	2.3 mg (15%)

Percent Daily Values are based on a 2,000 calorie diet. Your daily values may be higher or lower depending on your caloric needs.

FIBER-FILLED
BANANA COLADA SMOOTHIE

There is a belief that foods that grow from the same soil taste good when eaten together, and the combination of tropical pineapple and coconut validates this theory. These fruits have wonderfully complementary flavors, and they are both high in fiber, a necessary part of a healthy diet. Bananas are added for their creamy texture and because they are rich in potassium.

1 cup (235 ml) light coconut milk
1 cup (155 g) diced pineapple
1/3 cup (25 g) lightly packed shredded unsweetened coconut
1/4 cup (32 g) whey protein powder
2 tablespoons (30 g) bee pollen
1/2 teaspoon (2.5 ml) pure rum extract
2 cups (300 g) banana slices, frozen
2 tablespoons (6 g) grated coconut for garnish (optional)

▓ Combine coconut milk, pineapple, coconut, whey protein powder, bee pollen, and rum extract in a blender or smoothie maker. Blend on high speed for 45 seconds or until mixture is puréed and smooth. Add banana slices, and blend on high speed again until mixture is smooth. Serve immediately, garnished with grated coconut, if desired.

▓ **YIELD:** Four 1-cup (235-ml) servings

▓ **NUTRITIONAL ANALYSIS:** Each 1-cup serving provides 242 calories; 7 g total fat; 6 g saturated fat; 11 g protein; 38 g carbohydrate; 4 g dietary fiber; 18 mg cholesterol.

▓ **TIP:** A banana whose peel has turned black still has great flavor and sweetness, and if you find yourself with a bunch of extra-ripe bananas, do not despair. Purée the fruit and freeze it in ice cube trays. You are then set not only for making smoothies but also for baking banana bread or muffins at a moment's notice.

SUPERCHARGE NUTRIENTS:	% DAILY VALUE*
Vitamin A	117.6 IU (2%)
Vitamin B6	0.7 mg (36%)
Vitamin C	20.4 mg (34%)
Vitamin E	1.2 mg (6%)
Magnesium	48.1 mg (12%)
Manganese	0.9 mg (46%)
Selenium	2.2 mcg (3%)
Zinc	0.7 mg (5%)

* Percent Daily Values are based on a 2,000 calorie diet. Your daily values may be higher or lower depending on your caloric needs.

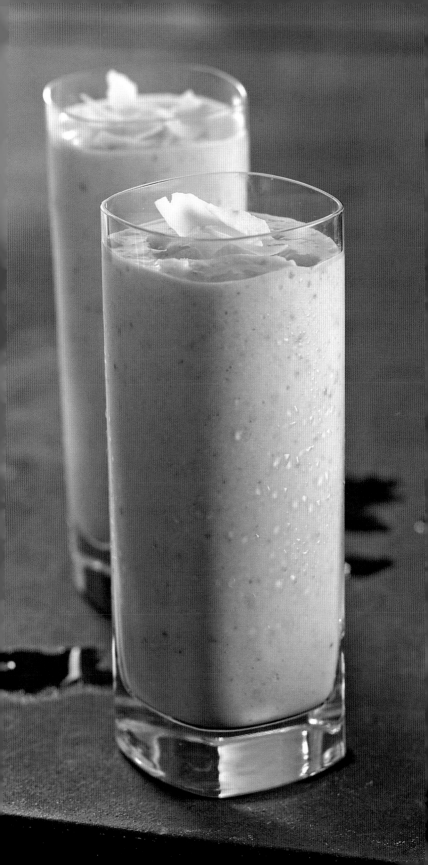

ANTIVIRAL VERVE
ORANGE COCONUT BANANA SMOOTHIE

Vitamin C is on the main line of defense against infection, and oranges are a great source of this vitamin. These succulent fruits also contain many flavonoids, which serve an important antioxidant function for your immune system. In addition to these benefits, the coconut in this recipe boosts immunity due to the fatty acid it contains, which is both antiviral and antibacterial.

2 navel oranges
$1/2$ cup (120 ml) silken tofu
$1/2$ cup (120 ml) light coconut milk
$1/2$ cup (120 ml) freshly squeezed orange juice
$1/2$ cup (40 g) lightly packed shredded unsweetened dried coconut
$1/4$ cup (80 g) fruit-only orange marmalade
$1/4$ cup (32 g) whey protein powder
2 tablespoons (30 g) bee pollen
2 cups (300 g) banana slices, frozen
4 orange segments for garnish (optional)

■ Peel oranges, then slice off white pith. Cut around sides of sections to release segments from remaining pith. Cut into $1/2$-inch (1-cm) dice.

■ Combine oranges, tofu, coconut milk, orange juice, coconut, orange marmalade, whey protein powder, and bee pollen in a blender or smoothie maker. Blend on high speed for 45 seconds or until mixture is puréed and smooth. Add banana slices, and blend on high speed again until mixture is smooth. Serve immediately, garnished with orange segments, if desired.

■ **YIELD:** Four 1-cup (235-ml) servings

■ **NUTRITIONAL ANALYSIS:** Each 1-cup serving provides 359 calories; 11 g total fat; 9 g saturated fat; 13 g protein; 57 g carbohydrate; 5 g dietary fiber; 18 mg cholesterol.

■ **TIP:** If you use sweetened coconut, pour boiling water over it and drain before adding it to the blender to remove much of the sugar.

SUPERCHARGE NUTRIENTS:	% DAILY VALUE*
Vitamin A	317.5 IU (6%)
Vitamin B6	0.5 mg (27%)
Vitamin C	65.2 mg (109%)
Vitamin E	1.2 mg (6%)
Magnesium	67.3 mg (17%)
Manganese	0.6 mg (28%)
Selenium	3.2 mcg (5%)
Zinc	1.1 mg (7%)

* Percent Daily Values are based on a 2,000 calorie diet. Your daily values may be higher or lower depending on your caloric needs.

B- AND C-RAISING
CRANBERRY ORANGE BANANA SMOOTHIE

Oranges and cranberries are a time-honored combination of sweet and tart flavors, and the creamy banana blends beautifully with them in this smoothie. All of these fruits are a boon to your immune system, with bananas strong in vitamin B6 and the other fruits full of vitamin C and flavonoids.

> 2 navel oranges
> 1 container (4 ounces or 112 g) plain low-fat yogurt
> 1/2 cup (120 ml) silken tofu
> 1/2 cup (150 g) cranberry sauce
> 1/4 cup (80 g) fruit-only orange marmalade
> 1/2 cup (50 g) fresh cranberries
> 1/4 cup (32 g) whey protein powder
> 2 tablespoons (30 g) bee pollen
> 2 cups (300 g) banana slices, frozen
> 4 orange segments for garnish (optional)

▩ Peel oranges, then slice off white pith. Cut around sides of sections to release segments from remaining pith. Cut into 1/2-inch (1-cm) dice.

▩ Combine oranges, yogurt, tofu, cranberry sauce, orange marmalade, cranberries, whey protein powder, and bee pollen in a blender or smoothie maker. Blend on high speed for 45 seconds or until mixture is puréed and smooth. Add banana slices, and blend on high speed again until mixture is smooth. Serve immediately, garnished with orange segments, if desired.

▩ **YIELD:** Four 1-cup (235-ml) servings

▩ **NUTRITIONAL ANALYSIS:** Each 1-cup serving provides 332 calories; 3 g total fat; 2 g saturated fat; 13 g protein; 68 g carbohydrate; 5 g dietary fiber; 23.5 mg cholesterol.

▩ **TIP:** I specify navel oranges for recipes because they are seedless, which speeds up prep time, and they are inherently sweet. If you cannot find them easily, it is always possible to use juice oranges; however, it is important to discard all of the pesky seeds.

SUPERCHARGE NUTRIENTS:	% DAILY VALUE*
Vitamin A	321.7 IU (6%)
Vitamin B6	0.5 mg (26%)
Vitamin C	52.2 mg (87%)
Vitamin E	1.1 mg (6%)
Magnesium	53.9 mg (13%)
Manganese	0.4 mg (20%)
Selenium	1.7 mcg (2%)
Zinc	0.9 mg (6%)

Percent Daily Values are based on a 2,000 calorie diet. Your daily values may be higher or lower depending on your caloric needs.

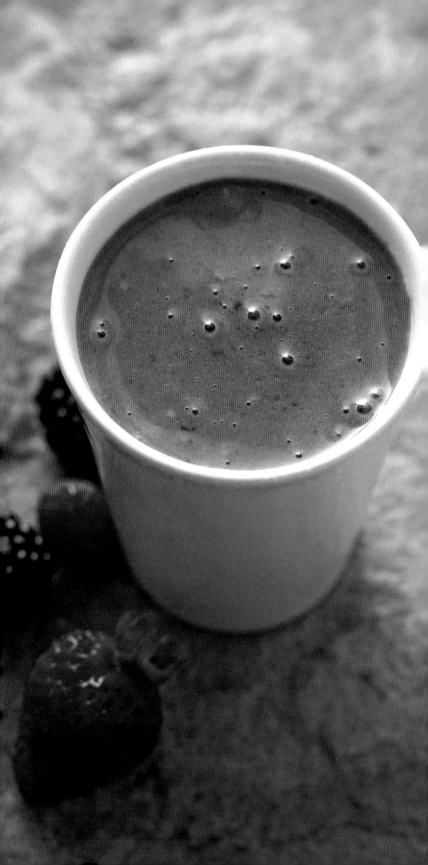

MARVELOUS MANGANESE VERY BERRY BANANA SMOOTHIE

Manganese is important for keeping bones healthy, so when flavorful raspberries and blackberries add their manganese-rich content to this nondairy smoothie—made creamy with bananas—it's a surefire winner.

1/2 cup (120 ml) plain soy milk
1/2 cup (120 ml) silken tofu
1/2 cup (70 g) blackberries
1/2 cup (60 g) raspberries
1/2 cup (85 g) strawberries, hulled and sliced
1/4 cup (32 g) whey protein powder
2 cups (300 g) banana slices, frozen
4 strawberry fans for garnish (optional)

▨ Combine soy milk, tofu, blackberries, raspberries, strawberries, and whey protein powder in a blender or smoothie maker. Blend on high speed for 45 seconds or until mixture is puréed and smooth. Add banana slices, and blend on high speed again until mixture is smooth. Serve immediately, garnished with strawberry fans, if desired.

▨ **YIELD:** Four 1-cup (235-ml) servings

▨ **NUTRITIONAL ANALYSIS:** Each 1-cup serving provides 183 calories; 2 g total fat; 1 g saturated fat; 10 g protein; 36 g carbohydrate; 4 g dietary fiber; 36 mg cholesterol.

▨ **TIP:** When selecting delicate berries like raspberries and blackberries, gently turn the package over to see if the paper blotter at the bottom of the carton is dry or has juice stains. A wet blotter indicates that the berries have either been bruised or are beginning to decay.

SUPERCHARGE NUTRIENTS:	% DAILY VALUE*
Vitamin A	225.7 IU (5%)
Vitamin B6	0.7 mg (35%)
Vitamin C	28.2 mg (47%)
Vitamin E	0.5 mg (3%)
Magnesium	53.7 mg (13%)
Manganese	0.7 mg (34%)
Selenium	3.2 mcg (5%)
Zinc	0.5 mg (3%)

* Percent Daily Values are based on a 2,000 calorie diet. Your daily values may be higher or lower depending on your caloric needs.

SUPER SELENIUM
BANANA BRAZIL NUT SMOOTHIE

Brazil nuts have about 2,500 times as much selenium as any other nut. Selenium is a trace mineral with powerful antioxidant properties that has been proven to protect against heart disease and prostate cancer. Brazil nuts are also full of magnesium, fiber, and zinc. Their buttery flavor melds beautifully with sweet, creamy bananas, which contribute vitamin B6 and other nutrients.

> 2 cups (300 g) chopped Brazil nuts
> 1 cup (235 ml) silken tofu
> 3 tablespoons (60 g) honey
> 2 tablespoons (30 ml) flaxseed oil
> ½ teaspoon (1.2 g) ground cinnamon, plus extra for garnish (optional)
> 2 cups (300 g) banana slices, frozen

▓ Preheat oven to 350°F (180°C, or gas mark 4). Place Brazil nuts on a baking sheet, and bake for 5 to 7 minutes or until lightly browned. Remove nuts from the oven, and allow to cool completely.

▓ Combine cooled nuts, tofu, honey, flaxseed oil, and cinnamon in a blender or smoothie maker. Blend on high speed for 45 seconds or until mixture is puréed and smooth. Add banana slices, and blend on high speed again until mixture is smooth. Serve immediately, garnished with a sprinkling of cinnamon, if desired.

▓ **YIELD:** Four 1-cup (235-ml) servings

▓ **NUTRITIONAL ANALYSIS:** Each 1-cup serving provides 547 calories; 25.5 g fat; 13 g protein; 69 g carbohydrate; 7 g dietary fiber; 0 mg cholesterol.

▓ **TIP:** While toasting nuts does not add to or diminish from their nutritional value, this step really enhances their flavor. Heating nuts releases aromatic and flavorful oils. These oils can also turn rancid, so it is best to store nuts in the freezer once they have been shelled.

SUPERCHARGE NUTRIENTS:	% DAILY VALUE*
Vitamin A	48.7 IU (1%)
Vitamin B6	0.5 mg (25%)
Vitamin C	6.8 mg (11%)
Vitamin E	7.4 mg (37%)
Magnesium	197.2 mg (49%)
Manganese	0.4 mg (19%)
Selenium	761.0 mcg (1087%)
Zinc	3.8 mg (25%)

Percent Daily Values are based on a 2,000 calorie diet. Your daily values may be higher or lower depending on your caloric needs.

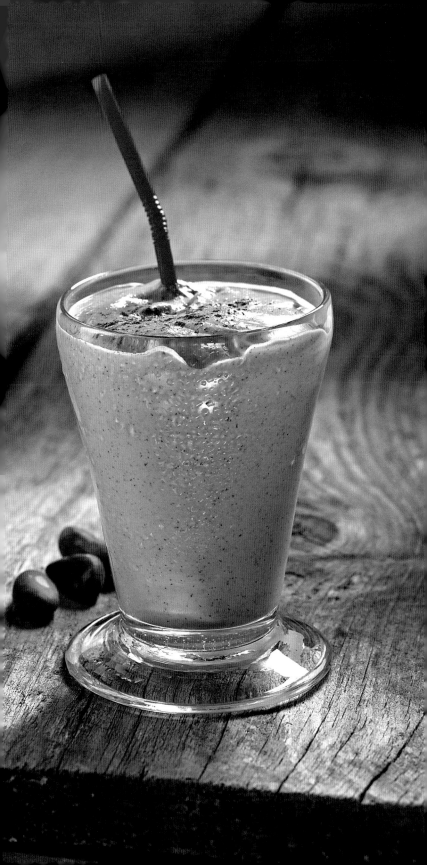

BLOOD PRESSURE PROUD
ALMOND FIG SMOOTHIE

Succulent figs, both in their fresh and dried forms, are an excellent source of potassium, a mineral that boosts your immune system and also helps to control blood pressure. Also a very good source of dietary fiber, these sweet fruits blend well with vitamin E-rich almonds for a thick and frosty drink.

1 container (8 ounces or 225 g) plain nonfat yogurt
1/2 cup (120 ml) silken tofu
1 cup (150 g) shelled almonds, not skinned
1 cup (150 g) dried figs, diced
1/2 cup (145 g) shelled sunflower seeds
1/4 cup (32 g) whey protein powder
2 tablespoons (30 g) bee pollen
1/2 teaspoon (1.2 g) ground cinnamon
1/2 teaspoon (2.5 ml) pure almond extract
5 fresh figs, stemmed, diced and frozen
4 dried figs for garnish (optional)

■ Combine yogurt, tofu, almonds, dried figs, sunflower seeds, whey protein powder, bell pollen, cinnamon, and almond extract in a blender or smoothie maker. Blend on high speed for 45 seconds or until mixture is puréed and smooth. Add figs, and blend on high speed again until mixture is smooth. Serve immediately, garnished with figs, if desired.

■ **YIELD:** Four 1-cup (235-ml) servings

■ **NUTRITIONAL ANALYSIS:** Each 1-cup serving provides 502 calories; 24 g total fat; 3 g saturated fat; 21 g protein; 58 g carbohydrate; 11.5 g dietary fiber; 20 mg cholesterol.

■ **TIP:** It was not too many years ago that fresh figs were virtually unknown in this country; even those grown in California and Florida were picked and then dried. Figs can vary more than most fruits in color; black mission are almost blackish-purple, while kadota are green and calimyrna are yellow. However, their flavor is almost identical.

SUPERCHARGE NUTRIENTS:	% DAILY VALUE*
Vitamin A	177.3 IU (4%)
Vitamin B6	0.3 mg (17%)
Vitamin C	6.4 mg (11%)
Vitamin E	10.1 mg (50%)
Magnesium	155.4 mg (39%)
Manganese	1.4 mg (69%)
Selenium	16.6 mcg (24%)
Zinc	3.0 mg (20%)

* Percent Daily Values are based on a 2,000 calorie diet. Your daily values may be higher or lower depending on your caloric needs.

C AND E-ASY
SPICED RASPBERRY ALMOND SMOOTHIE

This blushing pink smoothie has all the flavors of the classic Austrian dessert, the linzer torte, with a hint of cinnamon enlivening the sweet almonds and perky raspberries. The raspberries are packed with ellagic acid, a powerful antioxidant, as well as with vitamin C and dietary fiber, while the almonds add a high amount of vitamin E to the mix.

1 container (8 ounces or 225 g) raspberry low-fat yogurt
$^1/_2$ cup (120 ml) silken tofu
$^1/_2$ cup (75 g) shelled almonds, not skinned
$^1/_4$ cup (80 g) fruit-only raspberry preserves
$^1/_4$ cup (32 g) whey protein powder
2 tablespoons (30 g) bee pollen
$^1/_2$ teaspoon (1.2 g) ground cinnamon
2 cups (250 g) raspberries, frozen
Sprinkle of cinnamon for garnish (optional)

▓ Combine yogurt, tofu, almonds, raspberry preserves, whey protein powder, bee pollen, and cinnamon in a blender or smoothie maker. Blend on high speed for 45 seconds or until mixture is puréed and smooth. Add raspberries, and blend on high speed again until mixture is smooth. Serve immediately, garnished with a sprinkle of cinnamon, if desired.

▓ **YIELD:** Four 1-cup (235-ml) servings

▓ **NUTRITIONAL ANALYSIS:** Each 1-cup serving provides 352 calories; 8 g total fat; 1 g saturated fat; 14 g protein; 58 g carbohydrate; 8 g dietary fiber; 19.5 mg cholesterol.

▓ **TIP:** If you are out of almonds, then cashews are always the best substitute. Their flavor is equally sweet, and does not contain the assertive finish of walnuts or pecans.

SUPERCHARGE NUTRIENTS:	% DAILY VALUE*
Vitamin A	92.4 IU (2%)
Vitamin B6	0.1 mg (6%)
Vitamin C	26.9 mg (45%)
Vitamin E	1.6 mg (8%)
Magnesium	73.1 mg (18%)
Manganese	1.2 mg (60%)
Selenium	2.9 mcg (4%)
Zinc	1.6 mg (10%)

* Percent Daily Values are based on a 2,000 calorie diet. Your daily values may be higher or lower depending on your caloric needs.

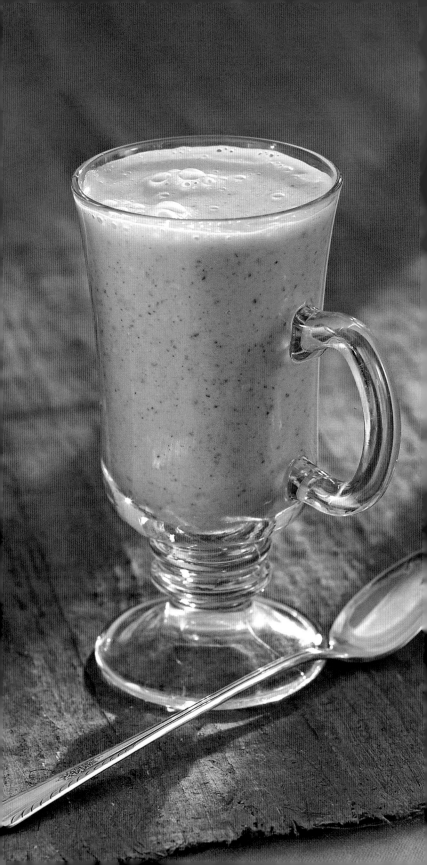

THROAT-SOOTHING
ALMOND HONEY BANANA SMOOTHIE

Opera singers swear by honey to soothe sore throats before perform-
ances. This smoothie harnesses that power and adds other ingredients—
such as manganese- and vitamin E-rich almonds—to boost the immune
system (and help cure that sore throat even faster).

> 1 container (8 ounces or 225 g) plain low-fat yogurt
> 1/2 cup (120 ml) silken tofu
> 1 cup (150 g) shelled almonds, not skinned
> 1/4 cup (85 g) honey
> 1/4 cup (32 g) whey protein powder
> 1/4 teaspoon (1.2 g) ground cinnamon
> 1/4 teaspoon (1.2 ml) pure vanilla extract
> 2 cups (300 g) banana slices, frozen
> Sprinkle of ground cinnamon for garnish (optional)

▨ Combine yogurt, tofu, almonds, honey, whey protein powder, cinnamon,
and vanilla extract in a blender or smoothie maker. Blend on high speed
for 45 seconds or until mixture is puréed and smooth. Add banana slices,
and blend on high speed again until mixture is smooth. Serve immediately,
garnished with a sprinkle of cinnamon, if desired.

▨ **YIELD:** Four 1-cup (235-ml) servings

▨ **NUTRITIONAL ANALYSIS:** Each 1-cup serving provides 446 calories; 19 g
total fat; 2 g saturated fat; 19 g protein; 57 g carbohydrate; 6 g dietary
fiber; 19.5 mg cholesterol.

▨ **TIP:** When sprinkling spices and herbs on foods as a garnish, the holes
in the spice jar may release more than you want. A useful method for
sprinkling just the right amount is to place the spice or herb in a fine
mesh strainer and tap it gently over the top of the food.

SUPERCHARGE NUTRIENTS:	% DAILY VALUE*
Vitamin A	113.4 IU (2%)
Vitamin B6	0.8 mg (38%)
Vitamin C	11.2 mg (19%)
Vitamin E	9.3 mg (47%)
Magnesium	147.9 mg (37%)
Manganese	1.2 mg (59%)
Selenium	7.8 mcg (11%)
Zinc	1.9 mg (13%)

*Percent Daily Values are based on a 2,000 calorie diet. Your daily values may be higher or
lower depending on your caloric needs.*

CHEERS FOR THE E-TEAM!
NUTTY ALMOND DATE SMOOTHIE

Both crunchy almonds and sunflower seeds are loaded with vitamin E, which protects cell membranes. The combination of succulent dried dates, sweet applesauce, and a bit of ginger balances the nutty richness with fruity sparkle.

2 cups (490 g) chilled unsweetened applesauce
1 cup (150 g) shelled almonds, not skinned
1/2 cup (145 g) shelled sunflower seeds
1/4 cup (32 g) whey protein powder
1/2 teaspoon (1 g) ground ginger
1/4 teaspoon (1.2 ml) pure almond extract
1 cup (175 g) firmly packed pitted dried dates
4 green tea ice cubes
Sprinkle of ground cinnamon or cinnamon stick for garnish (optional)

▨ Combine applesauce, almonds, sunflower seeds, whey protein powder, ginger, almond extract, and dates in a blender or smoothie maker. Blend on high speed for 45 seconds or until mixture is puréed and smooth. Add ice cubes, and blend on high speed again until mixture is smooth. Serve immediately, garnished with a sprinkle of cinnamon or cinnamon stick, if desired.

▨ **YIELD:** Four 1-cup (235-ml) servings

▨ **NUTRITIONAL ANALYSIS:** Each 1-cup serving provides 462 calories; 22 g total fat; 2 g saturated fat; 17 g protein; 58 g carbohydrate; 10.5 g dietary fiber; 19 mg cholesterol.

▨ **TIP:** Not only does it save time to keep the skins on the almonds but they also add health benefits. According to the *Journal of Nutrition*, the flavonoids in the skins team up with the vitamin E found in the nut meat to deliver a much stronger antioxidant punch.

SUPERCHARGE NUTRIENTS:	% DAILY VALUE*
Vitamin A	35.8 IU (3%)
Vitamin B6	0.3 mg (14%)
Vitamin C	17.1 mg (28%)
Vitamin E	9.0 mg (45%)
Magnesium	118.6 mg (30%)
Manganese	1.3 mg (64%)
Selenium	14.8 mcg (21%)
Zinc	1.9 mg (13%)

Percent Daily Values are based on a 2,000 calorie diet. Your daily values may be higher or lower depending on your caloric needs.

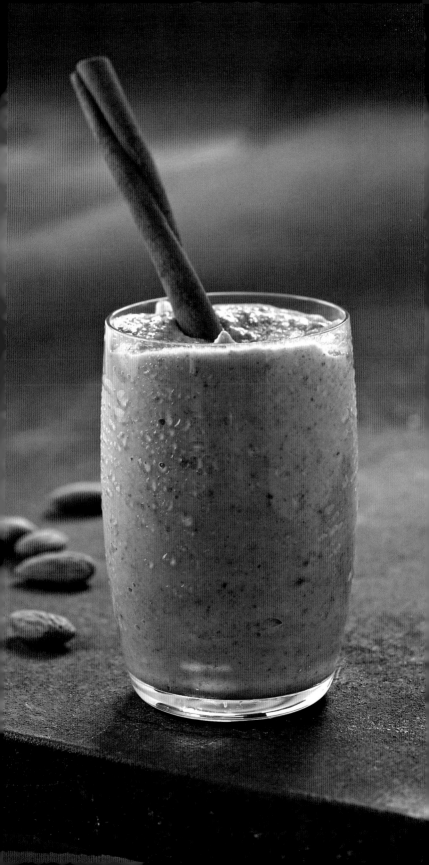

HEART-HEALTHY
APPLE WALNUT RAISIN SMOOTHIE

This smoothie, loaded with heart-healthy omega-3s, has all the traditional flavors of an apple pie—including the spices. The raisins contain boron, a trace mineral that prevents bone loss, especially in post-menopausal women. Apples are high in flavonoids with strong antioxidant powers.

1 cup (150 g) shelled walnuts
1 container (4 ounces or 112 g) vanilla low-fat yogurt
1 cup (245 g) chilled unsweetened applesauce
2 sweet eating apples (such as McIntosh or Red Delicious),
   cored and diced
$3/4$ cup (110 g) raisins
$1/4$ cup (32 g) whey protein powder
2 tablespoons (30 ml) flaxseed oil
$1/2$ teaspoon (1.2 g) apple pie spice
1 cup (140 g) vanilla frozen yogurt
2 tablespoons chopped walnuts for garnish (optional)

■ Preheat the oven to 350°F (180°C, or gas mark 4). Place walnuts on a baking sheet, and bake for 5 to 7 minutes or until lightly browned. Remove nuts from the oven, and allow to cool completely.

■ Combine walnuts, yogurt, applesauce, apples, raisins, whey protein powder, flaxseed oil, and apple pie spice in a blender or smoothie maker. Blend on high speed for 45 seconds or until mixture is puréed and smooth. Add frozen yogurt, and blend on high speed again until mixture is smooth. Serve immediately, garnished with chopped walnuts, if desired.

■ **YIELD:** Four 1-cup (235-ml) servings

■ **NUTRITIONAL ANALYSIS:** Each 1-cup serving provides 440 calories; 21 g total fat; 2 g saturated fat; 15 g protein; 55 g carbohydrate; 4 g dietary fiber; 25 mg cholesterol.

■ **TIP:** If the apples you are using are tart, such as Granny Smith, add 1 to 2 tablespoons of honey or pure maple syrup to this recipe to compensate.

SUPERCHARGE NUTRIENTS:	% DAILY VALUE*
Vitamin A	152.7 IU (3%)
Vitamin B6	0.3 mg (14%)
Vitamin C	10.6 mg (18%)
Vitamin E	2.5 mg (13%)
Magnesium	69.5 mg (17%)
Manganese	1.0 mg (49%)
Selenium	5.2 mcg (7%)
Zinc	1.2 mg (8%)

* Percent Daily Values are based on a 2,000 calorie diet. Your daily values may be higher or lower depending on your caloric needs.

UPPING THE IRON
MANGO MACADAMIA COCONUT SMOOTHIE

Hawaiian macadamia nuts, with their rich sweet flavor, are now easy to find, and this treat from the tropics is a good source of iron. When joined with mangoes, rich in both vitamin C and beta-carotene, this smoothie boosts your immune system and tastes like a vacation to a sunny climate.

1 container (4 ounces or 112 g) peach low-fat yogurt
$1/2$ cup (120 ml) mango nectar
$1/2$ cup (120 ml) light coconut milk
$3/4$ cup (110 g) roasted macadamia nuts
$1/2$ cup (40 g) lightly packed shredded unsweetened dried coconut
$1/4$ cup (32 g) whey protein powder
2 tablespoons (30 g) bee pollen
2 cups (350 g) diced mango, frozen
4 mango spears for garnish (optional)

▨ Combine yogurt, mango nectar, coconut milk, macadamia nuts, coconut, whey protein powder, and bee pollen in a blender or smoothie maker. Blend on high speed for 45 seconds or until mixture is puréed and smooth. Add mango, and blend on high speed again until mixture is smooth. Serve immediately, garnished with mango spears, if desired.

▨ **YIELD:** Four 1-cup (235-ml) servings

▨ **NUTRITIONAL ANALYSIS:** Each 1-cup serving provides 419 calories; 30 g total fat; 11.5 g saturated fat; 13 g protein; 31 g carbohydrate; 6 g dietary fiber; 19 mg cholesterol.

▨ **TIP:** If you have trouble finding fruit nectars, such as mango or papaya, in the juice section of your supermarket, try the aisle where the Hispanic foods are shelved. These drinks are very popular in Latin America, and chances are you will find cans of them there.

SUPERCHARGE NUTRIENTS:	% DAILY VALUE*
Vitamin A	3243.5 IU (65%)
Vitamin B6	0.2 mg (12%)
Vitamin C	31.9 mg (53%)
Vitamin E	2.5 mg (13%)
Magnesium	65.0 mg (16%)
Manganese	0.4 mg (22%)
Selenium	4.2 mcg (6%)
Zinc	1.2 mg (8%)

* Percent Daily Values are based on a 2,000 calorie diet. Your daily values may be higher or lower depending on your caloric needs.

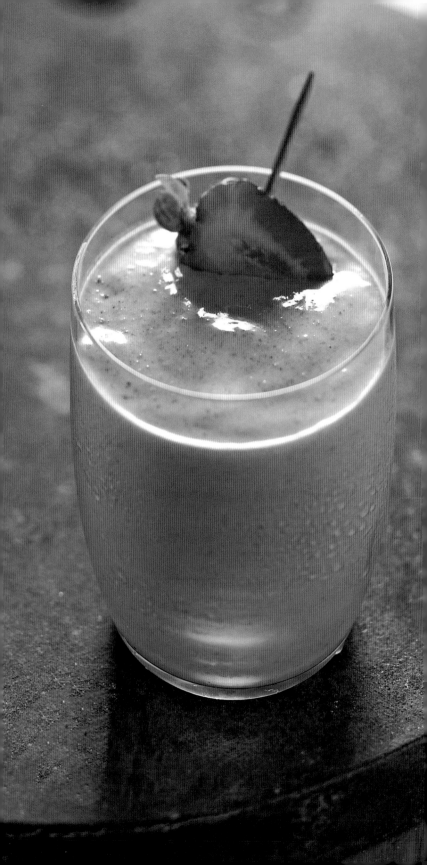

MANGANESE-E
STRAWBERRY ALMOND SMOOTHIE

It is not true that all fats are bad for your diet; the monounsaturated fat found in nuts, such as almonds, has been associated with a reduced risk of heart disease. Almonds are a great source of two minerals—manganese and magnesium—as well as vitamin E, and the vitamin C-rich strawberries add color and sweetness to this smoothie.

> 1 container (8 ounces or 225 g) strawberry low-fat yogurt
> 1/2 cup (120 ml) silken tofu
> 1/4 cup (80 g) fruit-only strawberry preserves
> 1 cup (150 g) shelled almonds, not skinned
> 1/4 cup (32 g) whey protein powder
> 2 tablespoons (30 ml) flaxseed oil
> 1 1/2 cups (220 g) strawberries, frozen
> 4 strawberry fans for garnish (optional)

■ Combine yogurt, tofu, strawberry preserves, almonds, whey protein powder, and flaxseed oil in a blender or smoothie maker. Blend on high speed for 45 seconds or until mixture is puréed and smooth. Add strawberries, and blend on high speed again until mixture is smooth. Serve immediately, garnished with strawberry fans, if desired.

■ **YIELD:** Four 1-cup (235-ml) servings

■ **NUTRITIONAL ANALYSIS:** Each 1-cup serving provides 461 calories; 27 g total fat; 2.5 g saturated fat; 17 g protein; 40.5 g carbohydrate; 5.5 g dietary fiber; 20 mg cholesterol.

■ **TIP:** If you like the taste of cream cheese but not its high fat content, you can give yogurt a firmer texture that resembles softened cream cheese, but that contains significantly less fat. To do so, place plain yogurt in a strainer lined with a paper coffee filter or a double layer of cheesecloth, and allow it to drain into a mixing bowl in the refrigerator for a minimum of 8 hours.

SUPERCHARGE NUTRIENTS:	% DAILY VALUE*
Vitamin A	55.6 IU (1%)
Vitamin B6	0.1 mg (4%)
Vitamin C	35.4 mg (59%)
Vitamin E	11.5 mg (58%)
Magnesium	151.4 mg (38%)
Manganese	1.2 mg (62%)
Selenium	4.1 mcg (6%)
Zinc	2.0 mg (13%)

* Percent Daily Values are based on a 2,000 calorie diet. Your daily values may be higher or lower depending on your caloric needs.

MINERAL MADNESS
CARROT, PINEAPPLE, BRAZIL NUT SMOOTHIE

Juicy pineapple is a great source of manganese, and buttery-flavored Brazil nuts are super-rich in selenium. So when you join them with the sweet flavor of carrot, you have minerals galore in a smoothie that tastes like a liquid version of carrot cake.

1 cup (150 g) chopped Brazil nuts
3/4 cup (175 ml) chilled carrot juice
1 medium carrot, scrubbed, and cut into 1/2-inch (1-cm) slices
1/3 cup (80 ml) silken tofu
1/4 cup (32 g) whey protein power
2 tablespoons (30 ml) flaxseed oil
3/4 teaspoon (1.5 g) ground cinnamon
1 1/2 cups (250 g) pineapple cubes, frozen
1/2 cup (70 g) vanilla frozen yogurt
4 pineapple spears for garnish (optional)

▓ Preheat oven to 350°F (180°C, or gas mark 4). Place Brazil nuts on a baking sheet, and bake for 5 to 7 minutes or until lightly browned. Remove nuts from oven, and allow to cool completely.

▓ Combine Brazil nuts, carrot juice, carrot, tofu, whey protein powder, flaxseed oil, and cinnamon in a blender or smoothie maker. Blend on high speed for 45 seconds or until mixture is puréed and smooth. Add pineapple and frozen yogurt, and blend on high speed again until mixture is smooth. Serve immediately, garnished with pineapple spears, if desired.

▓ **YIELD:** Four 1-cup (235-ml) servings

▓ **NUTRITIONAL ANALYSIS:** Each 1-cup serving provides 350 calories; 17 g total fat; 4 g saturated fat; 15 g protein; 36 g carbohydrate; 4 g dietary fiber; 36 mg cholesterol.

▓ **TIP:** While we think about spices and herbs as sources of flavor, always keep in mind that they are sources of nutrients, too. In this case the cinnamon adds a big dose of manganese to the smoothie's nutritional profile.

SUPERCHARGE NUTRIENTS:	% DAILY VALUE*
Vitamin A	6696.9 IU (134%)
Vitamin B6	0.2 mg (12%)
Vitamin C	12.9 mg (21%)
Vitamin E	5.4 mg (27%)
Magnesium	113.1 mg (28%)
Manganese	1.1 mg (56%)
Selenium	380.3 mcg (543%)
Zinc	1.9 mg (13%)

* Percent Daily Values are based on a 2,000 calorie diet. Your daily values may be higher or lower depending on your caloric needs.

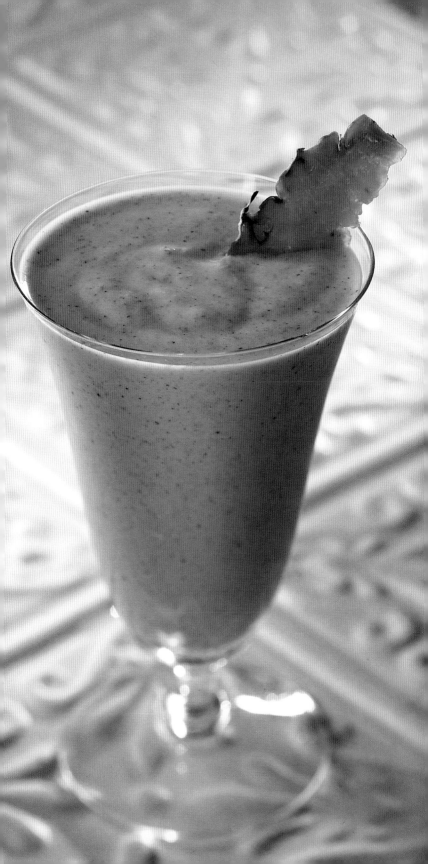

BUTTER-E RICH
ALMOND PEAR SMOOTHIE

Pears are a good source of dietary fiber as well as copper, a mineral that helps the body protect against free radical damage. Their subtle, buttery flavor blends wonderfully with vitamin-E rich almonds in this smoothie.

1 cup (235 ml) pear nectar

1/2 cup (120 ml) silken tofu

1 cup (150 g) shelled almonds, not skinned

1/2 cup (85 g) dried pears, diced

1/4 cup (32 g) whey protein powder

2 tablespoons (30 g) bee pollen

2 tablespoons (16 g) crystallized ginger

3 ripe pears, cored, diced, and frozen

1/2 cup (70 g) vanilla frozen yogurt

2 tablespoons finely chopped crystallized ginger for garnish (optional)

■ Combine pear nectar, tofu, almonds, dried pears, whey protein powder, bee pollen, and crystallized ginger in a blender or smoothie maker. Blend on high speed for 45 seconds or until mixture is puréed and smooth. Add pears and frozen yogurt, and blend on high speed again until mixture is smooth. Serve immediately, garnished with chopped crystallized ginger, if desired.

■ **YIELD:** Four 1-cup (235-ml) servings

■ **NUTRITIONAL ANALYSIS:** Each 1-cup serving provides 454 calories; 16 g total fat; 2 g saturated fat; 17 g protein; 65.5 g carbohydrate; 10 g dietary fiber; 34 mg cholesterol.

■ **TIP:** Pears are considered a mild fruit that can be tolerated by people who have problems digesting many fruits due to their inherent acidity. They can be eaten raw, or they are best cooked gently by poaching or baking.

SUPERCHARGE NUTRIENTS:	% DAILY VALUE*
Vitamin A	94.0 IU (2%)
Vitamin B6	0.1 mg (6%)
Vitamin C	11.4 mg (19%)
Vitamin E	2.1 mg (11%)
Magnesium	105.4 mg (26%)
Manganese	0.8 mg (42%)
Selenium	0.9 mcg (1%)
Zinc	1.7 mg (11%)

Percent Daily Values are based on a 2,000 calorie diet. Your daily values may be higher or lower depending on your caloric needs.

MAVEN FOR MITOCHONDRIA
ALMOND RASPBERRY SMOOTHIE

Manganese is an essential mineral to keep your immune system in top infection-fighting order as it is the principal antioxidant enzyme in the mitochondria, the cell's power producers. Both raspberries and almonds are good sources of this trace mineral, and their flavors blend deliciously in this smoothie.

1 container (8 ounces or 225 g) raspberry nonfat yogurt

1/2 cup (120 ml) silken tofu

1/4 cup (80 g) fruit-only raspberry preserves

1 cup (150 g) shelled almonds, not skinned

1/2 cup (145 g) shelled sunflower seeds

1/4 cup (32 g) whey protein powder

2 tablespoons (30 ml) flaxseed oil

1/4 teaspoon (1.2 ml) pure almond extract

1 1/2 cups (190 g) raspberries, frozen

12 raspberries skewered onto 4 toothpicks for garnish (optional)

Combine yogurt, tofu, raspberry preserves, almonds, sunflower seeds, whey protein powder, flaxseed oil, and almond extract in a blender or smoothie maker. Blend on high speed for 45 seconds or until mixture is puréed and smooth. Add raspberries, and blend on high speed again until mixture is smooth. Serve immediately, garnished with raspberries, if desired.

YIELD: Four 1-cup (235-ml) servings

NUTRITIONAL ANALYSIS: Each 1-cup serving provides 469 calories; 30 g total fat; 3 g saturated fat; 18 g protein; 36 g carbohydrate; 8 g dietary fiber; 20 mg cholesterol.

TIP: Almonds, especially when still in their skins, are one nut that does not benefit very much from toasting; that is why I omitted that step from most of the recipes that include them. If you fear your almonds are old, however, it is a good idea to toast them in a 350°F (180°C, or gas mark 4) oven for 5 to 7 minutes to release their flavor.

SUPERCHARGE NUTRIENTS:	% DAILY VALUE*
Vitamin A	108.5 IU (2%)
Vitamin B6	0.2 mg (11%)
Vitamin C	14.9 mg (25%)
Vitamin E	10.3 mg (52%)
Magnesium	129.4 mg (32%)
Manganese	1.4 mg (69%)
Selenium	16.2 mcg (23%)
Zinc	2.5 mg (17%)

* Percent Daily Values are based on a 2,000 calorie diet. Your daily values may be higher or lower depending on your caloric needs.

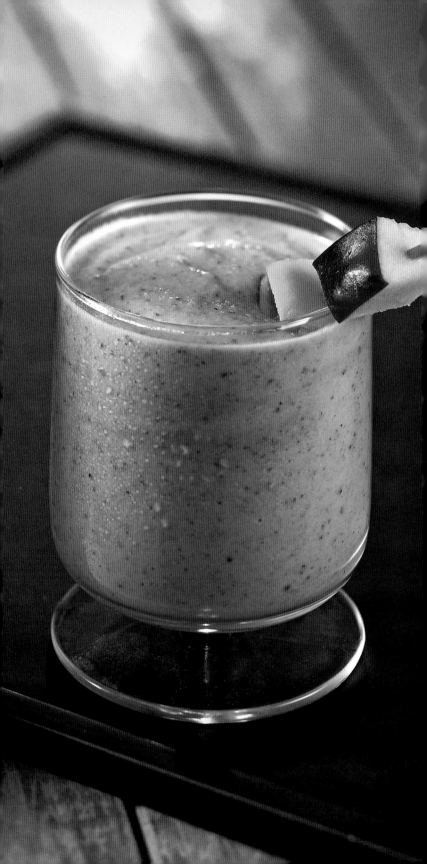

FIBER FANTASTIC
MAPLE DATE NUT SMOOTHIE

Maple syrup, like honey, adds nutrients as well as sweetness to smoothies. This thickened sap from maple trees contains manganese and zinc, both of which are necessary for a healthy immune system. Brazil nuts and dates are terrific sources of dietary fiber, and their richness marries well with the subtle flavor of apple in this smoothie.

   1 cup (235 ml) plain soy milk
   1/4 cup (60 ml) pure maple syrup
   1 cup (175 g) firmly packed pitted dried dates, diced
   3/4 cup (115 g) chopped Brazil nuts
   1 sweet eating apple (such as McIntosh or Red Delicious), cored,
      and diced
   1/4 cup (32 g) whey protein powder
   2 tablespoons (30 ml) flaxseed oil
   4 green tea ice cubes
   1/2 cup (70 g) vanilla frozen yogurt
   4 apple slices for garnish (optional)

▓ Combine soy milk, maple syrup, dates, Brazil nuts, apple, whey protein powder, and flaxseed oil in a blender or smoothie maker. Blend on high speed for 45 seconds or until mixture is puréed and smooth. Add ice cubes and frozen yogurt, and blend on high speed again until mixture is smooth. Serve immediately, garnished with apple slices, if desired.

▓ **YIELD:** Four 1-cup (235-ml) servings

▓ **NUTRITIONAL ANALYSIS:** Each 1-cup serving provides 472 calories; 16 g total fat; 3 g saturated fat; 14 g protein; 73 g carbohydrate; 6.5 g dietary fiber; 21 mg cholesterol.

▓ **TIP:** It has become much easier to find pure maple syrup at the supermarket. So make sure you see "pure" on the label and not "pancake syrup," which is nothing but corn syrup with added artificial maple flavor.

SUPERCHARGE NUTRIENTS:	% DAILY VALUE*
Vitamin A	206.5 IU (4%)
Vitamin B6	0.2 mg (9%)
Vitamin C	2.0 mg (3%)
Vitamin E	3.6 mg (18%)
Magnesium	98.0 mg (25%)
Manganese	0.8 mg (40%)
Selenium	504.3 mcg (720%)
Zinc	2.4 mg (16%)

Percent Daily Values are based on a 2,000 calorie diet. Your daily values may be higher or lower depending on your caloric needs.

HEALING HONEY
PEANUT BANANA SMOOTHIE

In addition to sweetening this smoothie, honey serves a role in boosting the immune system; It is one of the few sources of pinocembrin, an antioxidant. Honey is also a healing agent—during World War I, it was mixed with cod liver oil and used to dress wounds on the battlefield. It adds a wonderfully delicate flavor to this crunchy smoothie.

 1 cup (235 ml) plain soy milk
 1/2 cup (120 ml) silken tofu
 1/4 cup (85 g) honey
 1 cup (145 g) shelled peanuts
 1/4 cup (60 g) shelled sunflower seeds
 1/4 cup (32 g) whey protein powder
 1/2 teaspoon (1.2 g) ground cinnamon
 1/2 teaspoon (2.5 ml) pure vanilla extract
 2 cups (300 g) banana slices, frozen
 Sprinkling of cinnamon for garnish (optional)

■ Combine soy milk, tofu, honey, peanuts, sunflower seeds, whey protein powder, cinnamon, and vanilla extract in a blender or smoothie maker. Blend on high speed for 45 seconds or until mixture is puréed and smooth. Add banana slices, and blend on high speed again until mixture is smooth. Serve immediately, garnished with a sprinkling of cinnamon, if desired.

■ **YIELD:** Four 1-cup (235-ml) servings

■ **NUTRITIONAL ANALYSIS:** Each 1-cup serving provides 428 calories; 24 g total fat; 3.5 g saturated fat; 21 g protein; 40 g carbohydrate; 6 g dietary fiber; 18 mg cholesterol.

■ **TIP:** If your honey has crystallized and is almost impossible to spoon out, place the jar in a pan of very hot tap water for about ten minutes and it should become liquid again. Do not place the jar in the microwave, which can heat it too much.

SUPERCHARGE NUTRIENTS:	% DAILY VALUE*
Vitamin A	234.5 IU (5%)
Vitamin B6	0.8 mg (42%)
Vitamin C	10.6 mg (18%)
Vitamin E	7.0 mg (35%)
Magnesium	126.6 mg (32%)
Manganese	1.2 mg (59%)
Selenium	11.8 mcg (17%)
Zinc	3.2 mg (21%)

* Percent Daily Values are based on a 2,000 calorie diet. Your daily values may be higher or lower depending on your caloric needs.

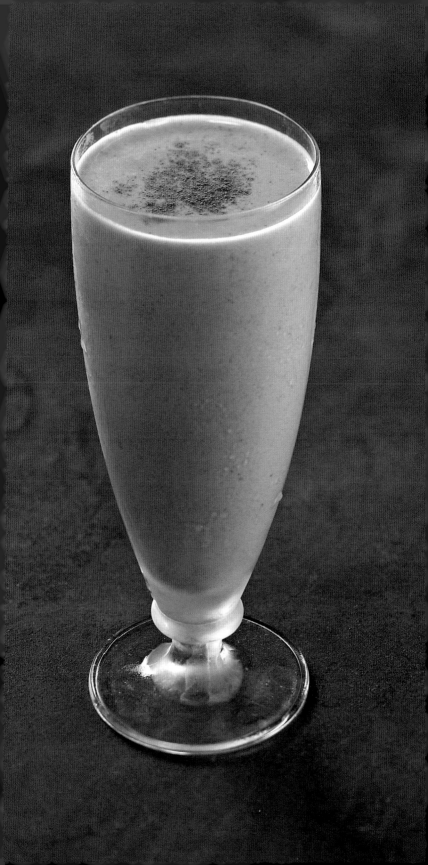

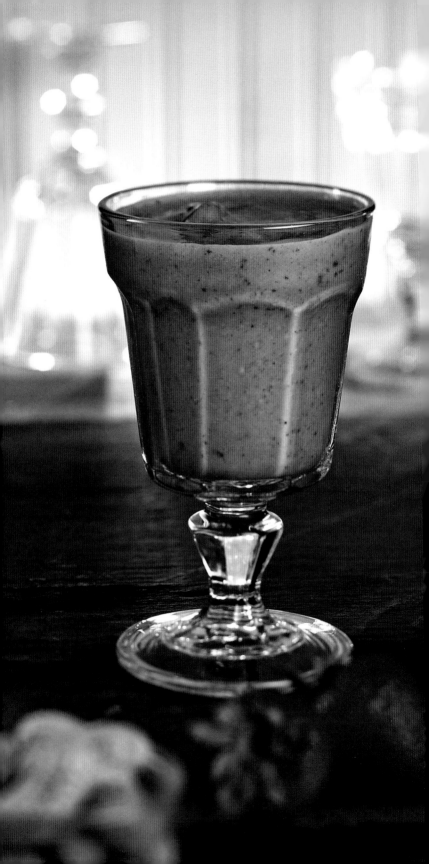

PROTEIN-POWERED PB&J SMOOTHIE

Contrary to their name, peanuts are actually a member of the legume family; they are botanically related to lentils and beans. They are a wonderful source of protein and contain high amounts of manganese and folate. Blended with vitamin C-rich strawberries, they create an excellent immune-boosting smoothie.

> 1 container (8 ounces or 225 g) strawberry low-fat yogurt
> 1 cup (235 ml) plain soy milk
> 1 cup (145 g) shelled peanuts
> 1/4 cup (32 g) whey protein powder
> 1/4 cup (80 g) fruit-only strawberry preserves
> 1 1/2 cups (220 g) strawberries, frozen
> 4 strawberry fans for garnish (optional)

▓ Combine yogurt, soy milk, peanuts, whey protein powder, and strawberry preserves in a blender or smoothie maker. Blend on high speed for 45 seconds or until mixture is puréed and smooth. Add strawberries, and blend on high speed again until mixture is smooth. Serve immediately, garnished with strawberry fans, if desired.

▓ **YIELD:** Four 1-cup (235-ml) servings

▓ **NUTRITIONAL ANALYSIS:** Each 1-cup serving provides 388 calories; 17 g total fat; 3 g saturated fat; 20 g protein; 39 g carbohydrate; 4 g dietary fiber; 20 mg cholesterol.

▓ **TIP:** If you're wondering how to select the best peanuts in their shells, pick one up and shake it, looking for two signs of quality. First, it should feel heavy for its size. Second, it should not rattle, since a rattling sound suggests that the peanut kernels have dried out. Furthermore, the shells should be free from cracks, dark spots, and insect damage.

SUPERCHARGE NUTRIENTS:	% DAILY VALUE*
Vitamin A	178.3 IU (4%)
Vitamin B6	0.1 mg (7%)
Vitamin C	36.7 mg (61%)
Vitamin E	2.9 mg (15%)
Magnesium	98.3 mg (25%)
Manganese	1.0 mg (49%)
Selenium	1.0 mcg (1%)
Zinc	3.0 mg (20%)

* Percent Daily Values are based on a 2,000 calorie diet. Your daily values may be higher or lower depending on your caloric needs.

REGULAR REGIME
VERY BERRY SMOOTHIE

Bright color is a sign that foods are high in antioxidant phytonutrients, and all berries with their tart and sweet flavor qualify. Berries are also good sources of dietary fiber, needed for your body's regularity. The whole really is better than the sum of its berry parts in this smoothie, as you will see when sipping the complex flavor of this drink.

> 1 container (8 ounces or 225 g) strawberry nonfat yogurt
> 1/2 cup (120 ml) cranberry juice
> 1/2 cup (120 ml) silken tofu
> 1/2 cup (75 g) strawberries
> 1/4 cup (32 g) whey protein powder
> 2 tablespoons (30 g) bee pollen
> 1 cup (145 g) blueberries, frozen
> 1 cup (145 g) blackberries, frozen
> 4 strawberry fans for garnish (optional)

▧ Combine yogurt, cranberry juice, tofu, strawberries, whey protein powder, and bee pollen in a blender or smoothie maker. Blend on high speed for 45 seconds or until mixture is puréed and smooth. Add blueberries and blackberries, and blend on high speed again until mixture is smooth. Serve immediately, garnished with strawberry fans, if desired.

▧ **YIELD:** Four 1-cup (235-ml) servings

▧ **NUTRITIONAL ANALYSIS:** Each 1-cup serving provides 158 calories; 2 g total fat; 1 g saturated fat; 13 g protein; 24 g carbohydrate; 4 g dietary fiber; 20 mg cholesterol.

▧ **TIP:** Berries are the easiest of all fruits to freeze. Rinse them, pat them dry with paper towels, and then arrange them on a baking sheet covered with a sheet of plastic wrap. They should be frozen solid within an hour, at which time they can be transferred to a heavy resealable plastic bag.

SUPERCHARGE NUTRIENTS:	% DAILY VALUE*
Vitamin A	141.9 IU (3%)
Vitamin B6	0.1 mg (5%)
Vitamin C	29.2 mg (49%)
Vitamin E	1.3 mg (6%)
Magnesium	40.7 mg (10%)
Manganese	0.5 mg (23%)
Selenium	2.0 mcg (3%)
Zinc	1.3 mg (8%)

* Percent Daily Values are based on a 2,000 calorie diet. Your daily values may be higher or lower depending on your caloric needs.

C-RAGEOUS
BLUEBERRY CITRUS SMOOTHIE

Vitamin C is your immune system's first line of defense in fighting infection, and all of the fruits in this smoothie are good sources of this vital nutrient, which must be eaten on a regular basis because it cannot be stored in the body. Blueberries are also touted as the fruit with the best antioxidant activity, so this smoothie is great—and delicious—protection for your body.

1 container (8 ounces or 225 g) lemon low-fat yogurt
1/2 cup (120 ml) freshly squeezed orange juice
1/4 cup (80 g) fruit-only orange marmalade
1/4 cup (32 g) whey protein powder
2 tablespoons (30 g) bee pollen
2 cups (290 g) blueberries
1 cup (140 g) lemon sorbet
4 orange slices for garnish (optional)

■ Combine yogurt, orange juice, orange marmalade, whey protein powder, bee pollen, and blueberries in a blender or smoothie maker. Blend on high speed for 45 seconds or until mixture is puréed and smooth. Add lemon sorbet, and blend on high speed again until mixture is smooth. Serve immediately, garnished with orange slices, if desired.

■ **YIELD:** Four 1-cup (235-ml) servings

■ **NUTRITIONAL ANALYSIS:** Each 1-cup serving provides 256 calories; 1 g total fat; 1 g saturated fat; 12 g protein; 52.5 g carbohydrate; 3.5 g dietary fiber; 20 mg cholesterol.

■ **TIP:** How much juice you can squeeze out of an orange depends on how you treat it before cutting it in half. Either roll it hard on the counter for a moment, or microwave it on high (100% power) for 30 seconds. Both of these techniques break down the fibers so the juice is easier to extract.

SUPERCHARGE NUTRIENTS:	% DAILY VALUE*
Vitamin A	290.2 IU (6%)
Vitamin B6	0.1 mg (6%)
Vitamin C	59.8 mg (100%)
Vitamin E	1.8 mg (9%)
Magnesium	31.6 mg (8%)
Manganese	0.3 mg (15%)
Selenium	2.2 mcg (3%)
Zinc	1.0 mg (7%)

* Percent Daily Values are based on a 2,000 calorie diet. Your daily values may be higher or lower depending on your caloric needs.

PURPLE GOLD
BLUEBERRY BLACKBERRY SMOOTHIE

Blackberries are a treasure trove of manganese and zinc, and when you complement those nutrients with the powerhouse of antioxidants in blueberries, your richly colored and richly flavored smoothie becomes as good for your health as it is to drink!

1 container (8 ounces or 225 g) blueberry low-fat yogurt
1 cup (235 ml) unsweetened purple grape juice
2 tablespoons (30 g) bee pollen
1 tablespoon (15 ml) freshly squeezed lemon juice
1 cup (145 g) blueberries, frozen
1 cup (145 g) blackberries, frozen
1/2 cup (70 g) vanilla frozen yogurt
12 blackberries or blueberries threaded onto 4 bamboo skewers for garnish (optional)

■ Combine yogurt, grape juice, bee pollen, and lemon juice in a blender or smoothie maker. Blend on high speed for 45 seconds or until mixture is puréed and smooth. Add blueberries, blackberries, and frozen yogurt, and blend on high speed again until mixture is smooth. Serve immediately, garnished with fruit skewers, if desired.

■ **YIELD:** Four 1-cup (235-ml) servings

■ **NUTRITIONAL ANALYSIS:** Each 1-cup serving provides 183 calories; 2 g total fat; 1 g saturated fat; 6 g protein; 38 g carbohydrate; 4 g dietary fiber; 4 mg cholesterol.

■ **TIP:** Many fruit recipes include a tablespoon or two of lemon or lime juice. The juice's tart flavor will not be noticed in the finished dish, and its presence perks the taste buds and actually makes the fruit's sweet flavors more pronounced.

SUPERCHARGE NUTRIENTS:	% DAILY VALUE*
Vitamin A	80.1 IU (2%)
Vitamin B6	0.1 mg (7%)
Vitamin C	8.4 mg (14%)
Vitamin E	1.3 mg (6%)
Magnesium	28.6 mg (7%)
Manganese	0.5 mg (26%)
Selenium	0.5 mcg (1%)
Zinc	0.9 mg (6%)

* Percent Daily Values are based on a 2,000 calorie diet. Your daily values may be higher or lower depending on your caloric needs.

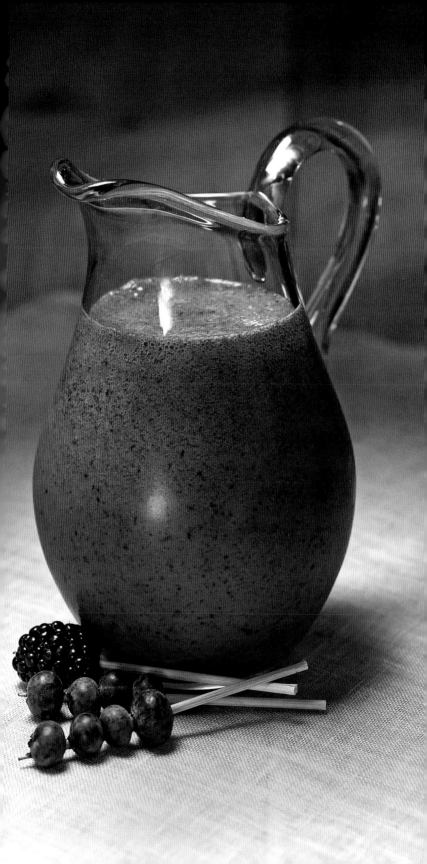

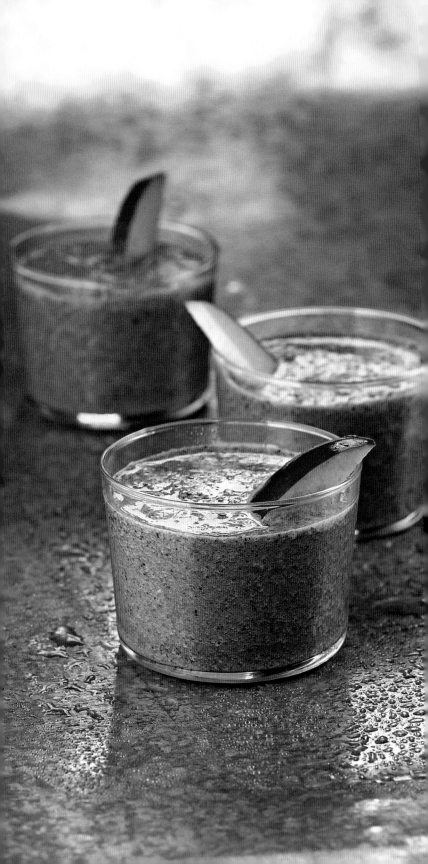

FLAVONOID FIESTA
APPLE BLUEBERRY SMOOTHIE

There is a synergistic relationship between flavonoids—the chemicals that give foods their color—and vitamin C: The flavonoids empower vitamin C to fight infection. Sweet apples and vibrant blueberries are both loaded with flavonoids, and when blended, they produce a luscious flavor and a lovely lavender color that make this smoothie a visually appealing taste treat.

1 container (8 ounces or 225 g) blueberry low-fat yogurt

$1/2$ cup (120 ml) chilled cloudy apple juice

1 sweet eating apple (such as McIntosh or Red Delicious), cored and diced

$1/4$ cup (32 g) whey protein powder

1 $1/2$ cups (220 g) blueberries, frozen

4 apple wedges for garnish (optional)

■ Combine yogurt, apple juice, apple, and whey protein powder in a blender or smoothie maker. Blend on high speed for 45 seconds or until mixture is puréed and smooth. Add blueberries, and blend on high speed again until mixture is smooth. Serve immediately, garnished with an apple wedge, if desired.

■ **YIELD:** Four 1-cup (235-ml) servings

■ **NUTRITIONAL ANALYSIS:** Each 1-cup serving provides 142 calories: 1 g total fat; 1 g saturated fat; 9 g protein; 25 g carbohydrate; 3 g dietary fiber; 20 mg cholesterol.

■ **TIP:** Never peel apples when making a smoothie, and try to avoid peeling them in general. The pigments in the skin contain quercitin, a powerful flavonoid.

SUPERCHARGE NUTRIENTS:	% DAILY VALUE*
Vitamin A	81.6 IU (2%)
Vitamin B6	0.09 mg (4%)
Vitamin C	4.1 mg (7%)
Vitamin E	0.8 mg (4%)
Magnesium	17.0 mg (4%)
Manganese	0.1 mg (7%)
Selenium	0.5 mcg (1%)
Zinc	0.4 mg (2%)

* Percent Daily Values are based on a 2,000 calorie diet. Your daily values may be higher or lower depending on your caloric needs.

DIVINE DETOX
BLUEBERRY GRAPEFRUIT SMOOTHIE

In addition to being high in infection-fighting vitamin C, grapefruit also contains phytonutrients called limonoids that help to detoxify the body.

   1 red or pink grapefruit
   1 container (8 ounces or 225 g) blueberry nonfat yogurt
   1/2 cup (120 ml) silken tofu
   1/2 cup (120 ml) freshly squeezed grapefruit juice
   1/4 cup (32 g) whey protein powder
   2 tablespoons (40 g) honey
   2 tablespoons (30 g) bee pollen
   2 cups (290 g) blueberries, frozen
   4 grapefruit segments for garnish (optional)

■ Peel grapefruit, then slice off white pith. Cut around sides of sections to release segments from remaining pith. Cut into 1/2-inch (1-cm) dice.

■ Combine grapefruit, yogurt, tofu, grapefruit juice, whey protein powder, honey, and bee pollen in a blender or smoothie maker. Blend on high speed for 45 seconds or until mixture is puréed and smooth. Add blueberries, and blend on high speed again until mixture is smooth. Serve immediately, garnished with grapefruit segments, if desired.

■ **YIELD:** Four 1-cup (235-ml) servings

■ **NUTRITIONAL ANALYSIS:** Each 1-cup serving provides 181 calories; 1 g total fat; 0.5 g saturated fat; 12 g protein; 34 g carbohydrate; 3 g dietary fiber; 20 mg cholesterol.

■ **TIP:** Once candied, leftover citrus peels make a great treat. To make, simmer the sliced peels in water for 20 minutes. Drain, and repeat this entire process twice more (using fresh water each time). Cover the drained peels with honey, and cook in a saucepan over a low flame for 10 to 15 minutes or until tender, stirring often. Remove the peels with a slotted spoon and roll each piece in granulated sugar (to keep them separate). Store at room temperature, tightly covered.

SUPERCHARGE NUTRIENTS:	% DAILY VALUE*
Vitamin A	275.3 IU (6%)
Vitamin B6	0.1 mg (5%)
Vitamin C	39.5 mg (66%)
Vitamin E	0.9 mg (5%)
Magnesium	35.3 mg (9%)
Manganese	0.3 mg (15%)
Selenium	2.8 mcg (4%)
Zinc	0.8 mg (5%)

* Percent Daily Values are based on a 2,000 calorie diet. Your daily values may be higher or lower depending on your caloric needs.

FREE RADICAL-FIGHTING
SPICED BLUEBERRY MANGO SMOOTHIE

Aromatic tropical mangoes are an excellent source of both vitamin C and beta-carotene, and their sweet flavor is the perfect foil to the somewhat tart blueberries in this smoothie. It is the blue-red pigment of blueberries that deliver a phytonutrient known as anthocyanidin, which neutralizes free radicals.

1 container (8 ounces or 225 g) blueberry nonfat yogurt
1/2 cup (120 ml) mango nectar
1 cup (145 g) blueberries
1/2 cup (145 g) shelled sunflower seeds
1/3 cup (85 g) mango chutney
1/4 cup (32 g) whey protein powder
2 tablespoons (30 ml) flaxseed oil
1 1/2 cups (210 g) mango cubes, frozen
4 mango spears for garnish (optional)

▓ Combine yogurt, mango nectar, blueberries, sunflower seeds, mango chutney, whey protein powder, and flaxseed oil in a blender or smoothie maker. Blend on high speed for 45 seconds or until mixture is puréed and smooth. Add mango cubes, and blend on high speed again until mixture is smooth. Serve immediately, garnished with mango spears, if desired.

▓ **YIELD:** Four 1-cup (235-ml) servings

▓ **NUTRITIONAL ANALYSIS:** Each 1-cup serving provides 327 calories; 15 g total fat; 2 g saturated fat; 13 g protein; 39 g carbohydrate; 4 g dietary fiber; 20 mg cholesterol.

▓ **TIP:** It is now quite easy to find chutney in supermarkets due to the growth of interest in Indian cuisine. But if you do not have it, here is a way to replicate its flavor: Combine 1/4 cup (75 g) of a fruit-only preserve with 2 tablespoons (30 ml) rice wine vinegar and a few drops of hot red pepper sauce.

SUPERCHARGE NUTRIENTS:	% DAILY VALUE*
Vitamin A	2629 IU (53%)
Vitamin B6	0.3 mg (14%)
Vitamin C	30.1 mg (50%)
Vitamin E	10.4 mg (52%)
Magnesium	52.7 mg (13%)
Manganese	0.5 mg (26%)
Selenium	15.0 mcg (21%)
Zinc	1.4 mg (10%)

* Percent Daily Values are based on a 2,000 calorie diet. Your daily values may be higher or lower depending on your caloric needs.

PROTEIN-PACKED
BERRY GOOD BLUEBERRY SMOOTHIE

Like most dairy products, cream cheese is a good source of vitamin A, calcium, and protein. When joined with blueberries, a stellar antioxidant, the result is a delicious drink that tastes like cheesecake.

1 container (8 ounces or 225 g) blueberry low-fat yogurt
1 package (3 ounces or 85 g) cream cheese, cut into $^1/_2$-inch
  (1-cm) pieces
$^1/_2$ cup (120 ml) silken tofu
$^1/_4$ cup (80 g) fruit-only blueberry preserves
$^1/_4$ cup (42 g) dried blueberries
$^1/_4$ cup (32 g) whey protein powder
2 $^1/_2$ cups (365 g) blueberries, frozen
16 blueberries threaded onto 4 bamboo skewers for garnish (optional)

▨ Combine yogurt, cream cheese, tofu, blueberry preserves, dried blueberries, and whey protein powder in a blender or smoothie maker. Blend on high speed for 45 seconds or until mixture is puréed and smooth. Add blueberries, and blend on high speed again until mixture is smooth. Serve immediately, garnished with blueberry skewers, if desired.

▨ **YIELD:** Four 1-cup (235-ml) servings

▨ **NUTRITIONAL ANALYSIS:** Each 1-cup serving provides 273 calories; 9 g total fat; 5 g saturated fat; 11 g protein; 38 g carbohydrate; 4 g dietary fiber; 42 mg cholesterol.

▨ **TIP:** If a sweetener is added to fruit-only preserves, it must be a fruit product, such as fructose, and not refined granulated sugar. This explains why these preserves are a better health choice for smoothies or for spreading on toast.

SUPERCHARGE NUTRIENTS:	% DAILY VALUE*
Vitamin A	408.0 IU (8%)
Vitamin B6	0.1 mg (6%)
Vitamin C	3.5 mg (6%)
Vitamin E	1.3 mg (6%)
Magnesium	22.9 mg (6%)
Manganese	0.2 mg (11%)
Selenium	3.2 mcg (5%)
Zinc	0.6 mg (4%)

* Percent Daily Values are based on a 2,000 calorie diet. Your daily values may be higher or lower depending on your caloric needs.

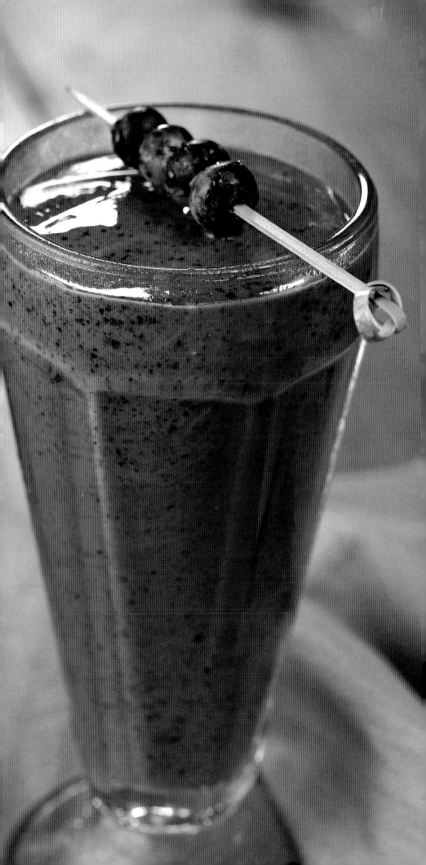

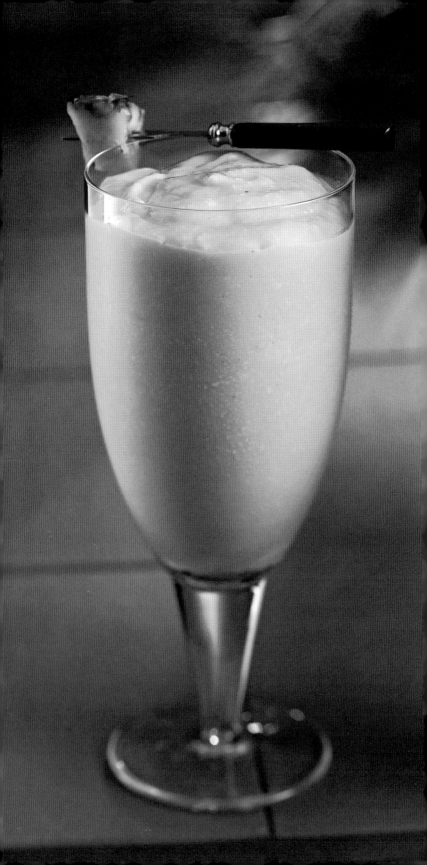

C-SUPER
MANGO PINEAPPLE SMOOTHIE

You can never get too much of the all-important antioxidant vitamin C. That said, it is best taken at various intervals throughout the day because your body excretes what it does not need at the moment, making it impossible to store any for the future. These two tropical treats—mango and pineapple—deliver plenty of this necessary nutrient.

1 container (8 ounces or 225 g) plain low-fat yogurt
1/2 cup (120 ml) silken tofu
1 1/2 cups (260 g) diced mango
1/2 cup (40 g) unsweetened dried shredded coconut
2 tablespoons (30 g) bee pollen
1/2 teaspoon (2.5 ml) pure coconut extract
1 cup (155 g) diced pineapple, frozen
4 pineapple or mango spears for garnish (optional)

■ Combine yogurt, tofu, mango, coconut, bee pollen, and coconut extract in a blender or smoothie maker. Blend on high speed for 45 seconds or until mixture is puréed and smooth. Add pineapple, and blend on high speed again until mixture is smooth. Serve immediately, garnished with pineapple spears, if desired.

■ **YIELD:** Four 1-cup (235-ml) servings

■ **NUTRITIONAL ANALYSIS:** Each 1-cup serving provides 183 calories; 7 g total fat; 5 g saturated fat; 6 g protein; 27 g carbohydrate; 4 g dietary fiber; 1 mg cholesterol.

■ **TIP:** Mangoes can be difficult to peel because their seed is elliptical and located somewhat off center in the fruit. The best way to slice a mango is to hold the fruit on its side and cut off the flesh from both sides of the seed. Then turn it over and cut the fruit away from the sides.

SUPERCHARGE NUTRIENTS:	% DAILY VALUE*
Vitamin A	2422.2 IU (48%)
Vitamin B6	0.2 mg (11%)
Vitamin C	27.5 mg (46%)
Vitamin E	1.5 mg (7%)
Magnesium	35.5 mg (9%)
Manganese	1.0 mg (48%)
Selenium	5.9 mcg (8%)
Zinc	1.1 mg (8%)

* Percent Daily Values are based on a 2,000 calorie diet. Your daily values may be higher or lower depending on your caloric needs.

THIAMIN-TOUTING PINEAPPLE ORANGE SMOOTHIE

While thiamin, also called vitamin B1, is not directly linked to the immune system, it is certainly important to maintain a good supply of energy for your body, and both pineapple and oranges are a good source of it. Along with the manganese in pineapple and vitamin C in oranges, this healthful smoothie will keep you in tip-top shape.

> 2 navel oranges
> 1/2 cup (120 ml) freshly squeezed orange juice
> 1/2 cup (120 ml) silken tofu
> 1/4 cup (32 g) whey protein powder
> 2 tablespoons (30 g) bee pollen
> 2 teaspoons (5 g) grated orange zest
> 2 cups (310 g) diced pineapple, frozen
> 4 orange segments or pineapple spears for garnish (optional)

■ Grate 2 teaspoons zest from oranges, and set aside. Peel oranges, then slice off white pith. Cut around sides of sections to release segments from remaining pith. Cut into 1/2-inch (1-cm) dice.

■ Combine oranges, orange juice, tofu, whey protein powder, bee pollen, and orange zest in a blender or smoothie maker. Blend on high speed for 45 seconds or until mixture is puréed and smooth. Add pineapple, and blend on high speed again until mixture is smooth. Serve immediately, garnished with orange segments, if desired.

■ **YIELD:** Four 1-cup (235-ml) servings

■ **NUTRITIONAL ANALYSIS:** Each 1-cup serving provides 151 calories; 1 g total fat; 1 g saturated fat; 11 g protein; 27 g carbohydrate; 4 g dietary fiber; 18 mg cholesterol.

■ **TIP:** The zest from citrus fruit is what adds an aromatic component to any dish in which they are included. This colored portion of the peel is where all of the aromatic oils are located, and your nose begins to enjoy a dish before your taste buds ever come into contact with the food.

SUPERCHARGE NUTRIENTS:	% DAILY VALUE*
Vitamin A	236.5 IU (5%)
Vitamin B6	0.2 mg (9%)
Vitamin C	92.8 mg (155%)
Vitamin E	0.7 mg (4%)
Magnesium	30.5 mg (8%)
Manganese	0.9 mg (47%)
Selenium	0.1 mcg (0%)
Zinc	0.6 mg (4%)

* Percent Daily Values are based on a 2,000 calorie diet. Your daily values may be higher or lower depending on your caloric needs.

SUNNY C
ORANGE DATE SMOOTHIE

In addition to their high vitamin C content, oranges are also an excellent source of a phytonutrient called hesperidin, which has been shown to reduce high blood pressure in some animals (studies have not been done on humans as yet). The sweet tangy flavor of the oranges is balanced by the mellow dates in this richly flavored smoothie.

2 navel oranges
3/4 cup (180 ml) freshly squeezed orange juice
1 tablespoon (15 ml) freshly squeezed lemon juice
1 cup (175 g) firmly packed pitted dried dates
1/4 cup (80 g) fruit-only orange marmalade
1/4 cup (32 g) whey protein powder
2 tablespoons (30 g) bee pollen
3/4 cup (105 g) orange sherbet
4 orange segments for garnish (optional)

▓ Peel oranges, then slice off white pith. Cut around sides of sections to release segments from remaining pith. Cut into 1/2-inch (1-cm) dice.

▓ Combine oranges, orange juice, lemon juice, dates, orange marmalade, whey protein powder, and bee pollen in a blender or smoothie maker. Blend on high speed for 45 seconds or until mixture is puréed and smooth. Add orange sherbet, and blend on high speed again until mixture is smooth. Serve immediately, garnished with orange segments, if desired.

▓ **YIELD:** Four 1-cup (235-ml) servings

▓ **NUTRITIONAL ANALYSIS:** Each 1-cup serving provides 322 calories; 2 g total fat; 1 g saturated fat; 11 g protein; 72 g carbohydrate; 6.5 g dietary fiber; 18 mg cholesterol.

▓ **TIP:** When you are measuring a dried fruit like pitted dates or dried apricots always push them down firmly into the measuring cup. Depending on the size of the pieces there can be a significant amount of air in the cup if they are loosely packed.

SUPERCHARGE NUTRIENTS:	% DAILY VALUE*
Vitamin A	278.7 IU (6%)
Vitamin B6	0.2 mg (9%)
Vitamin C	66.4 mg (111%)
Vitamin E	0.8 mg (4%)
Magnesium	40.9 mg (10%)
Manganese	0.1 mg (7%)
Selenium	2.2 mcg (3%)
Zinc	0.8 mg (5%)

Percent Daily Values are based on a 2,000 calorie diet. Your daily values may be higher or lower depending on your caloric needs.

TROPICAL TEAMWORK
PAPAYA PINEAPPLE SMOOTHIE

Pineapple, the fruit with the highest content of manganese, is a good source of vitamin C, and papaya is almost over-the-top when it comes to its vitamin-C level. Together, these two fruits add up to a delicious smoothie.

> 1 container (8 ounces or 225 g) plain low-fat yogurt
> 1/2 cup (120 ml) silken tofu
> 1/2 cup (120 ml) chilled papaya nectar
> 2 tablespoons (30 g) bee pollen
> 1 cup (140 g) diced papaya
> 1 1/2 cups (225 g) peach slices, frozen
> 4 pineapple spears for garnish (optional)

■ Combine yogurt, tofu, papaya nectar, bee pollen, and papaya in a blender or smoothie maker. Blend on high speed for 45 seconds or until mixture is puréed and smooth. Add peach slices, and blend on high speed again until mixture is smooth. Serve immediately, garnished with pineapple spears, if desired.

■ **YIELD:** Four 1-cup (235-ml) servings

■ **NUTRITIONAL ANALYSIS:** Each 1-cup serving provides 123 calories; 1 g total fat; 0 g saturated fat; 6 g protein; 24 g carbohydrate; 3 g dietary fiber; 1 mg cholesterol.

■ **TIP:** Pineapple may qualify as a super-food, but it cannot be used raw in gelatin desserts. It contains an enzyme that prevents the gelatin from thickening properly. Once processed for canning, however, it can be used.

SUPERCHARGE NUTRIENTS:	% DAILY VALUE*
Vitamin A	1089.5 IU (22%)
Vitamin B6	0.1 mg (5%)
Vitamin C	31.1 mg (52%)
Vitamin E	1.4 mg (7%)
Magnesium	25.6 mg (6%)
Manganese	0.1 mg (5%)
Selenium	4.1 mcg (6%)
Zinc	1.1 mg (7%)

Percent Daily Values are based on a 2,000 calorie diet. Your daily values may be higher or lower depending on your caloric needs.

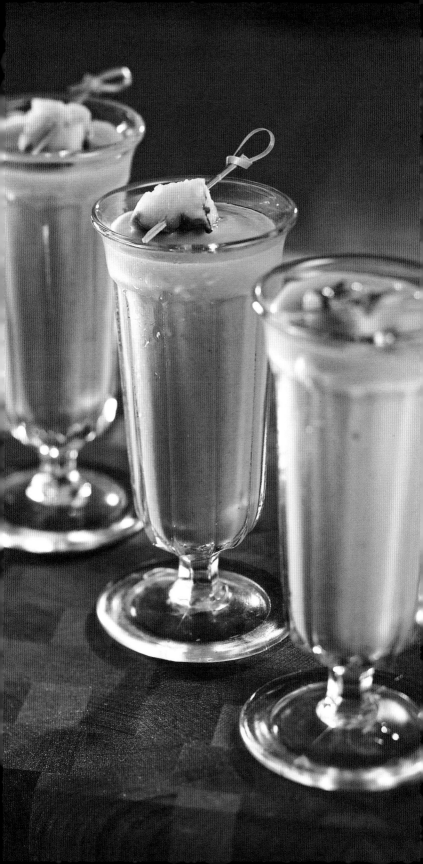

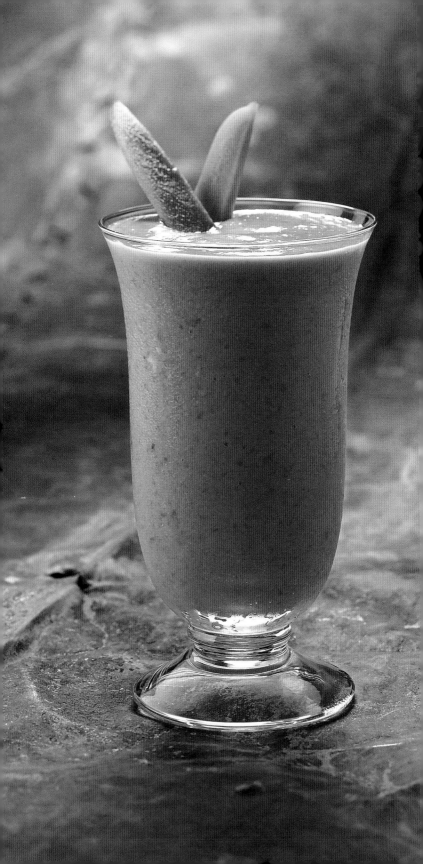

CUP OF COPPER
SESAME PAPAYA SMOOTHIE

Sesame seeds are a great source of copper, a nutrient we need to help our bodies utilize iron and fight free radicals. The subtle sesame flavor melds wonderfully with vitamin C-rich papaya in this smoothie.

> 1 cup (235 ml) chilled papaya nectar
> 1/2 cup (120 ml) silken tofu
> 1/3 cup (80 g) tahini
> 2 tablespoons (30 g) bee pollen
> 2 cups (350 g) diced papaya, frozen
> 4 papaya spears for garnish (optional)

▨ Combine papaya nectar, tofu, tahini, and bee pollen in a blender or smoothie maker. Blend on high speed for 45 seconds or until mixture is puréed and smooth. Add papaya pieces, and blend on high speed again until mixture is smooth. Serve immediately. Garnish with papaya spears, if desired.

▨ **YIELD:** Four 1-cup (235-ml) servings

▨ **NUTRITIONAL ANALYSIS:** Each 1-cup serving provides 136 calories; 5 g total fat; 1 g saturated fat; 4 g protein; 21 g carbohydrate; 3 g dietary fiber; 0 mg cholesterol.

▨ **TIP:** Save the skin when you peel a papaya and add it to a marinade for meat or poultry. Both the skin and flesh of this tropical treat contain papain, an enzyme that acts as a natural meat tenderizer.

SUPERCHARGE NUTRIENTS:	% DAILY VALUE*
Vitamin A	1483.4 IU (30%)
Vitamin B6	0.1 mg (3%)
Vitamin C	48.9 mg (81%)
Vitamin E	3.1 mg (15%)
Magnesium	27.8 mg (7%)
Manganese	0.1 mg (6%)
Selenium	0.5 mcg (1%)
Zinc	0.9 mg (6%)

Percent Daily Values are based on a 2,000 calorie diet. Your daily values may be higher or lower depending on your caloric needs.

LIVELY LIMONOIDS
SPICED PAPAYA GRAPEFRUIT SMOOTHIE

Vitamin C-rich grapefruit, which is also high in limonoids (phytonutrients that help form detoxifying enzymes), blends beautifully with sweet papaya in this lucious smoothie. From its color, you can guess that papaya is high in beta-carotene, which your body converts to vitamin A. Papaya is also a good source of vitamin E.

2 red or pink grapefruit
$1/2$ cup (120 ml) papaya nectar
$1/2$ cup (120 ml) silken tofu
$1/4$ cup (65 g) mango chutney
$1/4$ cup (32 g) whey protein powder
2 tablespoons (30 g) bee pollen
2 $1/2$ cups (440 g) diced papaya, frozen
4 papaya spears for garnish (optional)

Peel grapefruit, then slice off white pith. Cut around sides of sections to release segments from remaining pith. Cut into $1/2$-inch (1-cm) dice.

Combine grapefruit, papaya nectar, tofu, chutney, whey protein powder, and bee pollen in a blender or smoothie maker. Blend on high speed for 45 seconds or until mixture is puréed and smooth. Add papaya, and blend on high speed again until mixture is smooth. Serve immediately, garnished with papaya spears, if desired.

YIELD: Four 1-cup (235-ml) servings

NUTRITIONAL ANALYSIS: Each 1-cup serving provides 177 calories; 1 g total fat; 1 g saturated fat; 11 g protein; 33 g carbohydrate; 4 g dietary fiber; 18 mg cholesterol.

TIP: When selecting grapefruit, look for ones that feel heavy for their size; a heavy grapefruit will contain more juice. Another tip for picking the best is to examine the rind carefully. It should be smooth and finely textured; that is a tip that the fruit was allowed to ripen fully.

SUPERCHARGE NUTRIENTS:	% DAILY VALUE*
Vitamin A	2239.4 IU (45%)
Vitamin B6	0.1 mg (6%)
Vitamin C	107.1 mg (178%)
Vitamin E	2.0 mg (10%)
Magnesium	33.7 mg (8%)
Manganese	0.02 mg (1%)
Selenium	2.4 mcg (3%)
Zinc	0.7 mg (5%)

* Percent Daily Values are based on a 2,000 calorie diet. Your daily values may be higher or lower depending on your caloric needs.

INFECTION-FIGHTING
PAPAYA STRAWBERRY SMOOTHIE

Dietary fiber is crucial to your body to keep it running properly, and both strawberries and papaya are high in fiber. In addition, strawberries are high in polyphenols that are powerful antioxidants, and both fruits are an excellent source of infection-fighting vitamin C.

1 container (8 ounces or 225 g) strawberry low-fat yogurt
$^1/_2$ cup (120 ml) silken tofu
$^1/_4$ cup (80 g) fruit-only strawberry preserves
$^1/_4$ cup (32 g) whey protein powder
2 tablespoons (30 g) bee pollen
1 cup (145 g) strawberries
2 cups (350 g) diced papaya, frozen
4 strawberry fans for garnish (optional)

■ Combine yogurt, tofu, strawberry preserves, whey protein powder, bee pollen, and strawberries in a blender or smoothie maker. Blend on high speed for 45 seconds or until mixture is puréed and smooth. Add papaya, and blend on high speed again until mixture is smooth. Serve immediately, garnished with strawberry fans, if desired.

■ **YIELD:** Four 1-cup (235-ml) servings

■ **NUTRITIONAL ANALYSIS:** Each 1-cup serving provides 196 calories; 2 g total fat; 1 g saturated fat; 13 g protein; 34 g carbohydrate; 3 g dietary fiber; 20 mg cholesterol.

■ **TIP:** Especially early in the season, many strawberries can have tough white cores that are best removed. An easy way to accomplish this task is with a plastic drinking straw. Push it through the pointed end of the berry, and it will remove both the core and the green top at the other side.

SUPERCHARGE NUTRIENTS:	% DAILY VALUE*
Vitamin A	1463.2 IU (29%)
Vitamin B6	0.1 mg (4%)
Vitamin C	70.7 mg (118%)
Vitamin E	1.4 mg (7%)
Magnesium	39.5 mg (10%)
Manganese	0.2 mg (10%)
Selenium	2.7 mcg (4%)
Zinc	1.1 mg (7%)

Percent Daily Values are based on a 2,000 calorie diet. Your daily values may be higher or lower depending on your caloric needs.

CACHE OF CATECHINS
GREEN TEA PAPAYA SMOOTHIE

A study published in the *Journal of Allergy and Clinical Immunology* found that the antioxidants found in green tea are more effective than either vitamin C or vitamin E at protecting cells and DNA from free-radical damage. In this smoothie, green tea's flavor forms a subtle background for the vivid tropical taste of mineral-rich papaya.

- 1/2 cup (120 ml) chilled papaya nectar
- 1 tablespoon (15 ml) freshly squeezed lime juice
- 2 cups (350 g) diced papaya
- 1/4 cup (32 g) whey protein powder
- 2 tablespoons (30 g) bee pollen
- 8 green tea ice cubes
- 4 papaya and 4 lime wedges for garnish (optional)

■ Combine papaya nectar, lime juice, papaya, whey protein powder, and bee pollen in a blender or smoothie maker. Blend on high speed for 45 seconds or until mixture is puréed and smooth. Add ice cubes, and blend on high speed again until mixture is smooth. Serve immediately, garnished with papaya spears, if desired.

■ **YIELD:** Four 1-cup (235-ml) servings

■ **NUTRITIONAL ANALYSIS:** Each 1-cup serving provides 108 calories; 1 g total fat; 1 g saturated fat; 9 g protein; 17 g carbohydrate; 2 g dietary fiber; 18 mg cholesterol.

■ **TIP:** Tea should be brewed in small batches, and the leaves should always be removed immediately after the brewing time has elapsed. Rinse a ceramic pot with very hot water and place two tablespoons of tea leaves inside. Add three cups of boiling water, and stir gently. Allow the tea to steep for one minute, and then strain it into the tea pot from which it will be served. Leaves can be used again for a second pot of tea.

SUPERCHARGE NUTRIENTS:	% DAILY VALUE*
Vitamin A	1470.4 IU (29%)
Vitamin B6	0.05 mg (2%)
Vitamin C	51.0 mg (85%)
Vitamin E	1.4 mg (7%)
Magnesium	15.5 mg (4%)
Manganese	0.01 mg (1%)
Selenium	0.4 mcg (1%)
Zinc	0.5 mg (3%)

* Percent Daily Values are based on a 2,000 calorie diet. Your daily values may be higher or lower depending on your caloric needs.

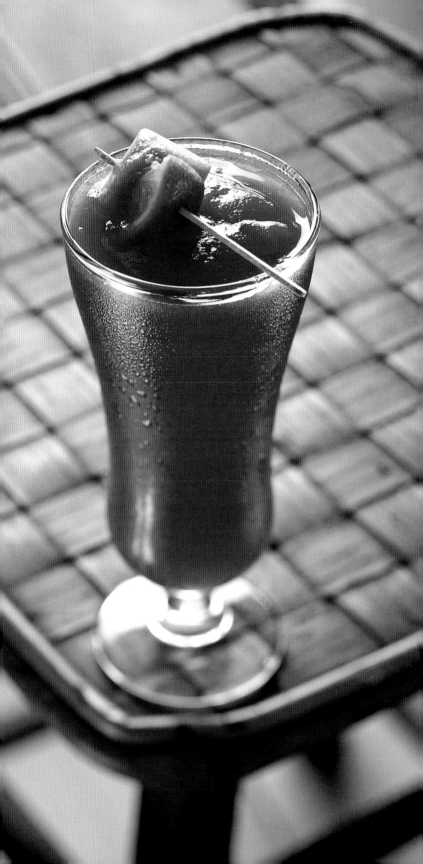

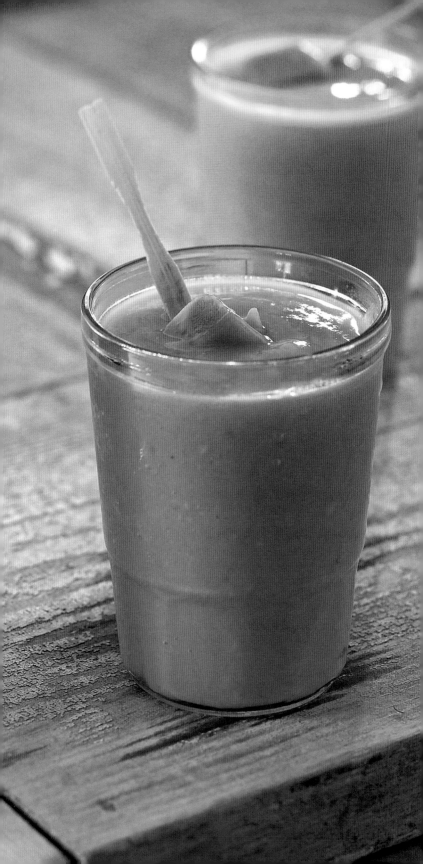

TENDER FOR THE TUMMY
GINGER PAPAYA SMOOTHIE

Ginger contains valuable minerals, including potassium, magnesium, and copper, and has many curative properties: It calms the stomach, mitigates nausea, and has anti-inflammatory properties that help with arthritis pain. It also adds fantastic flavor to this smoothie made with vitamin C- and folate-filled papaya.

1 cup (235 ml) chilled papaya nectar
1 container (8 ounces or 225 g) peach low-fat yogurt
1/2 cup (120 ml) silken tofu
1/4 cup (32 g) whey protein powder
3 tablespoons (24 g) crystallized ginger
2 cups (280 g) papaya cubes, frozen
4 papaya spears for garnish (optional)

■ Combine papaya nectar, yogurt, tofu, whey protein powder, and crystallized ginger in a blender or smoothie maker. Blend on high speed for 45 seconds or until mixture is puréed and smooth. Add papaya cubes, and blend on high speed again until mixture is smooth. Serve immediately, garnished with papaya spears, if desired.

■ **YIELD:** Four 1-cup (235-ml) servings

■ **NUTRITIONAL ANALYSIS:** Each 1-cup serving provides 174 calories; 1 g total fat; 1 g saturated fat; 10 g protein; 32 g carbohydrate; 2 g dietary fiber; 20 mg cholesterol.

■ **TIP:** Crystallized ginger is fresh ginger that has been cooked in sugar syrup to render it both sweet and tender. It is usually then coated with sugar to prevent the slices from sticking together. To find crystallized ginger, look in the baking section of your supermarket rather than the produce aisle.

SUPERCHARGE NUTRIENTS:	% DAILY VALUE*
Vitamin A	1528.4 IU (31%)
Vitamin B6	0.1 mg (3%)
Vitamin C	46.0 mg (77%)
Vitamin E	0.8 mg (4%)
Magnesium	24.2 mg (6%)
Manganese	0.1 mg (4%)
Selenium	2.0 mcg (3%)
Zinc	0.5 mg (4%)

* Percent Daily Values are based on a 2,000 calorie diet. Your daily values may be higher or lower depending on your caloric needs.

DANDY FOR DIGESTION
MINTED CANTALOUPE APPLE SMOOTHIE

While we may like mint for its fresh aroma and flavor, it also has been used for centuries as an herb to help digestion. The flavor of mint is a wonderful accent to the mild tastes of cantaloupe, a cache of beta-carotene, and apples.

> 1 container (8 ounces or 225 g) vanilla nonfat yogurt
> 1/2 cup (125 g) unsweetened applesauce
> 1/2 cup (120 ml) silken tofu
> 2 sweet eating apples (such as McIntosh or Red Delicious), cored and diced
> 2 sprigs fresh mint
> 2 tablespoons (30 ml) flaxseed oil
> 1 1/2 cups (235 g) diced cantaloupe, frozen
> 4 mint sprigs for garnish (optional)

■ Combine yogurt, applesauce, tofu, apples, mint, and flaxseed oil in a blender or smoothie maker. Blend on high speed for 45 seconds or until mixture is puréed and smooth. Add cantaloupe cubes, and blend on high speed again until mixture is smooth. Serve immediately, garnished with mint sprigs, if desired.

■ **YIELD:** Four 1-cup (235-ml) servings

■ **NUTRITIONAL ANALYSIS:** Each 1-cup serving provides 175 calories; 7 g total fat; 0.8 g saturated fat; 5 g protein; 15 g carbohydrate; 1 g dietary fiber; 2 mg cholesterol.

■ **TIP:** While some food authorities say that a cantaloupe with a well-developed netting on its rind tend to be riper, I have found that a better test is to shake the cantaloupe. A ripe melon will have juice in the cavity and you will be able to hear or feel it slosh around.

SUPERCHARGE NUTRIENTS:	% DAILY VALUE*
Vitamin A	1975.8 IU (40%)
Vitamin B6	0.1 mg (4%)
Vitamin C	26.0 mg (43%)
Vitamin E	1.3 mg (6%)
Magnesium	27.5 mg (7%)
Manganese	0.1 mg (4%)
Selenium	2.1 mcg (3%)
Zinc	0.7 mg (5%)

Percent Daily Values are based on a 2,000 calorie diet. Your daily values may be higher or lower depending on your caloric needs.

A-PLUS SPICED
CANTALOUPE PEACH SMOOTHIE

The sweet and hot elements of chutney add complexity to the flavor of this vivid orange smoothie, made with two fruits touted for a high concentration of vitamin A (which helps to boost your immune system). Peaches add a richness to the gentler flavor of the cantaloupe.

1 container (8 ounces or 225 g) peach nonfat yogurt
1 cup (155 g) diced cantaloupe
1/3 cup (85 g) mango chutney
1/4 cup (32 g) whey protein powder
2 tablespoons (30 g) bee pollen
2 cups (340 g) peach slices, frozen
1/2 cup (70 g) vanilla frozen yogurt
4 peach slices for garnish (optional)

▨ Combine yogurt, cantaloupe, chutney, whey protein powder, and bee pollen in a blender or smoothie maker. Blend on high speed for 45 seconds or until mixture is puréed and smooth. Add peach slices and frozen yogurt, and blend on high speed again until mixture is smooth. Serve immediately, garnished with peach slices, if desired.

▨ **YIELD:** Four 1-cup (235-ml) servings

▨ **NUTRITIONAL ANALYSIS:** Each 1-cup serving provides 171 calories; 2 g total fat; 1 g saturated fat; 13 g protein; 28 g carbohydrate; 3 g dietary fiber; 22.5 mg cholesterol.

▨ **TIP:** The traditional way to peel peaches calls for dropping them into boiling water for 30 seconds, and then refreshing them in ice water to allow the skins to slip off easily. There are new vegetable peelers on the market, however, that are fitted with serrated blades. These gadgets turn peeling both peaches and tomatoes into fast and simple tasks.

SUPERCHARGE NUTRIENTS:	% DAILY VALUE*
Vitamin A	2347.4 IU (47%)
Vitamin B6	0.1 mg (6%)
Vitamin C	28.7 mg (48%)
Vitamin E	1.4 mg (7%)
Magnesium	34.8 mg (9%)
Manganese	0.1 mg (5%)
Selenium	2.1 mcg (3%)
Zinc	1.1 mg (7%)

* Percent Daily Values are based on a 2,000 calorie diet. Your daily values may be higher or lower depending on your caloric needs.

MULTI-MINERAL
CANTALOUPE BLACKBERRY SMOOTHIE

Blackberries share many antioxidant qualities with their visual cousin, the blueberry, but they are also an excellent source of such important immune-boosting minerals as magnesium, manganese, and zinc. When combined with low-calorie cantaloupe, which is loaded with vitamin A and vitamin C, you have a very healthful and delicious smoothie.

> 1 container (8 ounces or 225 g) vanilla low-fat yogurt
> 1/2 cup (120 ml) silken tofu
> 2 cups (310 g) diced cantaloupe
> 1/4 cup (80 g) fruit-only blackberry preserves
> 1/4 cup (32 g) whey protein power
> 1 1/2 cups (220 g) blackberries, frozen
> 4 blackberries for garnish (optional)

■ Combine yogurt, tofu, cantaloupe, blackberry preserves, and whey protein powder in a blender or smoothie maker. Blend on high speed for 45 seconds or until mixture is puréed and smooth. Add blackberries, and blend on high speed again until mixture is smooth. Serve immediately, garnished with berry skewers, if desired.

■ **YIELD:** Four 1-cup (235-ml) servings

■ **NUTRITIONAL ANALYSIS:** Each 1-cup serving provides 202 calories; 2 g total fat; 1 g saturated fat; 11 g protein; 37 g carbohydrate; 4 g dietary fiber; 22 mg cholesterol.

■ **TIP:** Look for plump, fresh-looking blackberries packed in small containers, since they crush very easily. Do not wash blackberries before storing, as the moisture stimulates the growth of mold on the fruit. Blackberries are highly perishable and should be used within three days of picking or purchase.

SUPERCHARGE NUTRIENTS:	% DAILY VALUE*
Vitamin A	2686.6 IU (54%)
Vitamin B6	0.135 mg (7%)
Vitamin C	45.9 mg (60%)
Vitamin E	0.9 mg (5%)
Magnesium	35.7 mg (9%)
Manganese	0.8 mg (4%)
Selenium	2.6 mcg (4%)
Zinc	0.7 mg (4%)

* Percent Daily Values are based on a 2,000 calorie diet. Your daily values may be higher or lower depending on your caloric needs.

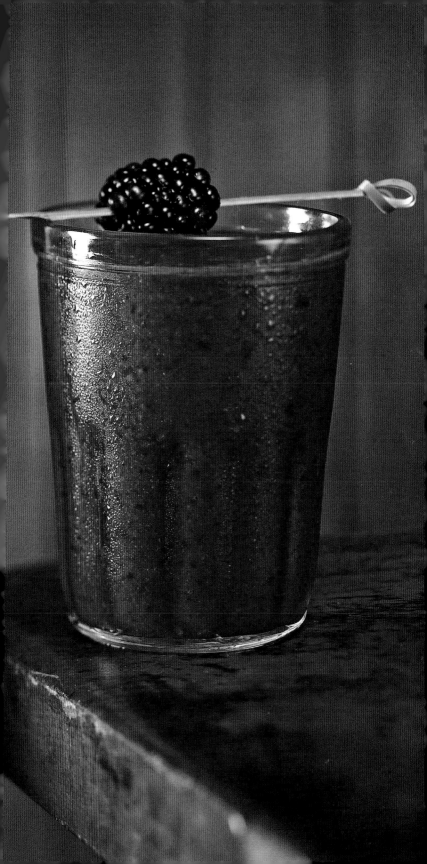

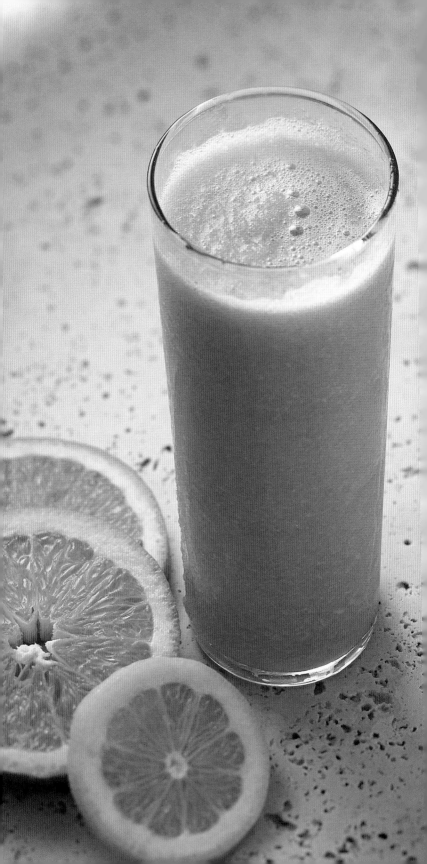

C-POWER
CANTALOUPE CITRUS SMOOTHIE

One whole cantaloupe delivers more vitamin A and vitamin C than you need in an entire day—talk about food superstar! When its rich flavor is joined with the sparkle of other vitamin C-rich citrus fruits like grapefruit and orange, your smoothie is armed and ready to protect you from harm.

- 1 cup (235 ml) freshly squeezed orange juice
- 1/2 cup (120 ml) freshly squeezed grapefruit juice, preferably from a red grapefruit
- 1/4 cup (32 g) whey protein powder
- 2 tablespoons (30 g) bee pollen
- 1 tablespoon (15 ml) freshly squeezed lemon or lime juice
- 2 cups (320 g) cantaloupe cubes, frozen
- 4 orange slices for garnish (optional)

▓ Combine orange juice, grapefruit juice, whey protein powder, bee pollen, and lemon or lime juice in a blender or smoothie maker. Blend on high speed for 20 seconds or until mixture is puréed and smooth. Add cantaloupe cubes, and blend on high speed again until mixture is smooth. Serve immediately, garnished with orange slices, if desired.

▓ **YIELD:** Four 1-cup (235-ml) servings

▓ **NUTRITIONAL ANALYSIS:** Each 1-cup serving provides 124 calories; 1 g total fat; 1 g saturated fat; 10 g protein; 20 g carbohydrate; 1 g dietary fiber; 18 mg cholesterol.

▓ **TIP:** Cantaloupe is a super-food and super healthy, but there have been cases of salmonella that resulted from bacteria being transferred from the melon's rind to its flesh when the melon was cut. Always wash a cantaloupe with warm soapy water before cutting it, and avoid buying pre-cut melons at the supermarket.

SUPERCHARGE NUTRIENTS:	% DAILY VALUE*
Vitamin A	2722.4 IU (54%)
Vitamin B6	0.2 mg (8%)
Vitamin C	80.1 mg (133%)
Vitamin E	0.8 mg (4%)
Magnesium	26.5 mg (7%)
Manganese	0.04 mg (2%)
Selenium	0.4 mcg (1%)
Zinc	0.6 mg (4%)

* Percent Daily Values are based on a 2,000 calorie diet. Your daily values may be higher or lower depending on your caloric needs.

E-XCELLENT
ORANGE ALMOND SMOOTHIE

This smoothie is inspired by famed cookbook author Claudia Roden's Middle Eastern almond and orange cake; the freshness of the orange flavor is accentuated by the sweetness of the almonds, which are high in heart-healthy monounsaturated fat as well as vitamin E. The vitamin C from the various forms of oranges adds its own boost to your immune system.

> 4 navel oranges
> 1 cup (150 g) shelled almonds, not skinned
> 1/2 cup (120 ml) freshly squeezed orange juice
> 1/2 cup (120 ml) silken tofu
> 1/2 cup (145 g) shelled sunflower seeds
> 1/4 cup (80 g) fruit-only orange marmalade
> 1/4 cup (32 g) whey protein powder
> 6 ice cubes made from freshly squeezed orange juice
> 4 orange segments for garnish (optional)

▓ Peel oranges, then slice off white pith. Cut around sides of sections to release segments from remaining pith. Cut into 1/2 -inch (1-cm) dice.

▓ Combine oranges, almonds, orange juice, tofu, sunflower seeds, orange marmalade, and whey protein powder in a blender or smoothie maker. Blend on high speed for 45 seconds or until mixture is puréed and smooth. Add ice cubes, and blend on high speed again until mixture is smooth. Serve immediately, garnished with orange segments, if desired.

▓ **YIELD:** Four 1-cup (235-ml) servings

▓ **NUTRITIONAL ANALYSIS:** Each 1-cup serving provides 476 calories; 28 g total fat; 3 g saturated fat; 20 g protein; 46 g carbohydrate; 9 g dietary fiber; 18 mg cholesterol.

▓ **TIP:** It is a misconception that nuts in their shells cannot turn rancid; they do turn rancid but they do it more slowly than once they are shelled. The best way to preserve nuts is to shell them and then place them in heavy, resealable plastic bags. They can be frozen successfully for up to a year.

SUPERCHARGE NUTRIENTS:	% DAILY VALUE*
Vitamin A	309.2 IU (6%)
Vitamin B6	0.3 mg (15%)
Vitamin C	94.2 mg (157%)
Vitamin E	17.1 mg (85%)
Magnesium	149.2 mg (37%)
Manganese	1.3 mg (65%)
Selenium	13.8 mcg (20%)
Zinc	2.3 mg (16%)

* Percent Daily Values are based on a 2,000 calorie diet. Your daily values may be higher or lower depending on your caloric needs.

ANTIOXIDANT ADVANTAGE
BERRY ORANGE SMOOTHIE

There's no question that a daily quotient of vitamin C is necessary to fight off infection; that's why drinking orange juice—especially if it is freshly-squeezed—is a great way to jump start your immune system in the morning. In this smoothie the bright flavor of oranges is joined by antioxidant-rich raspberries and cranberry sauce to give the drink a blushing pink color.

> 4 navel oranges
> 1 cup (235 ml) silken tofu
> 1/2 cup (160 g) fruit-only orange marmalade
> 1/2 cup (150 g) cranberry sauce
> 1/4 cup (32 g) whey protein powder
> 2 tablespoons (30 ml) flaxseed oil
> 1 1/2 cups (190 g) raspberries, frozen
> 4 orange segments for garnish (optional)

■ Peel oranges, then slice off white pith. Cut around sides of sections to release segments from remaining pith. Cut into 1/2 -inch (1-cm) dice.

▨ Combine oranges, tofu, orange marmalade, cranberry sauce, whey protein powder, and flaxseed oil in a blender or smoothie maker. Blend on high speed for 45 seconds or until mixture is puréed and smooth. Add raspberries, and blend on high speed again until mixture is smooth. Serve immediately, garnished with orange segments, if desired.

▨ **YIELD:** Four 1-cup (235-ml) servings

▨ **NUTRITIONAL ANALYSIS:** Each 1-cup serving provides 421 calories; 8 g total fat; 1 g saturated fat; 11 g protein; 83 g carbohydrate; 8 g dietary fiber; 18 mg cholesterol.

▨ **TIP:** It seems like a shame to waste the aromatic oils found in the orange zest, so take a few moments to grate it off before beginning this recipe. Make sure that you do not get any of the bitter white pith, and then freeze the zest for up to three months. It can be used in myriad ways.

SUPERCHARGE NUTRIENTS:	% DAILY VALUE*
Vitamin A	406.0 IU (8%)
Vitamin B6	0.1 mg (6%)
Vitamin C	86.1 mg (143%)
Vitamin E	2.0 mg (10%)
Magnesium	36.7 mg (9%)
Manganese	0.7 mg (34%)
Selenium	1.4 mcg (2%)
Zinc	0.5 mg (3%)

* Percent Daily Values are based on a 2,000 calorie diet. Your daily values may be higher or lower depending on your caloric needs.

C-PRISINGLY DELICIOUS
CITRUS STRAWBERRY SMOOTHIE

Sweet and sour flavors balance one another well in this smoothie filled with vitamin C-rich fruits. The drink's nutritional profile is further enhanced by including sunflower seeds, which have little effect on the flavor but add a large amount of vitamin E to the mix.

   2 navel oranges
   1 red grapefruit
   1 cup (235 ml) freshly squeezed orange juice
   2/3 cup (150 ml) freshly squeezed grapefruit juice, preferably
      from a red grapefruit
   1/2 cup (160 g) fruit-only strawberry preserves
   1/3 cup (75 g) shelled sunflower seeds
   1/4 cup (32 g) whey protein powder
   1 1/2 cups (220 g) strawberries, frozen
   4 fresh whole strawberries or strawberry fans for garnish (optional)

▨ Peel oranges and grapefruit, and slice off white pith. Cut around sides of sections to release segments from remaining pith. Cut into 1/2-inch (1-cm) dice.

▨ Combine oranges, grapefruit, orange juice, grapefruit juice, strawberry preserves, sunflower seeds, and whey protein powder in a blender or smoothie maker. Blend on high speed for 45 seconds or until mixture is puréed and smooth. Add strawberries, and blend on high speed again until mixture is smooth. Serve immediately, garnished with strawberry fans, if desired.

▨ **YIELD:** Four 1-cup (235-ml) servings

▨ **NUTRITIONAL ANALYSIS:** Each 1-cup serving provides 329 calories; 6 g total fat; 1 g saturated fat; 11 g protein; 62 g carbohydrate; 6 g dietary fiber; 18 mg cholesterol.

▨ **TIP:** If possible, always buy red rather than white grapefruit. The reason is found in the color: Red grapefruit contain far more carotenoids than their pale cousins.

SUPERCHARGE NUTRIENTS:	% DAILY VALUE*
Vitamin A	490.4 IU (10%)
Vitamin B6	0.2 mg (11%)
Vitamin C	137.4 mg (229%)
Vitamin E	5.9 mg (30%)
Magnesium	50.9 mg (13%)
Manganese	0.5 mg (25%)
Selenium	11.0 mcg (16%)
Zinc	0.9 mg (6%)

* Percent Daily Values are based on a 2,000 calorie diet. Your daily values may be higher or lower depending on your caloric needs.

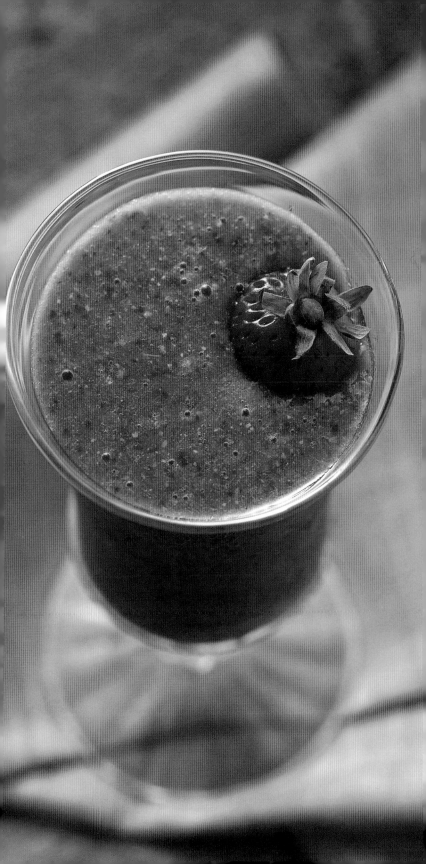

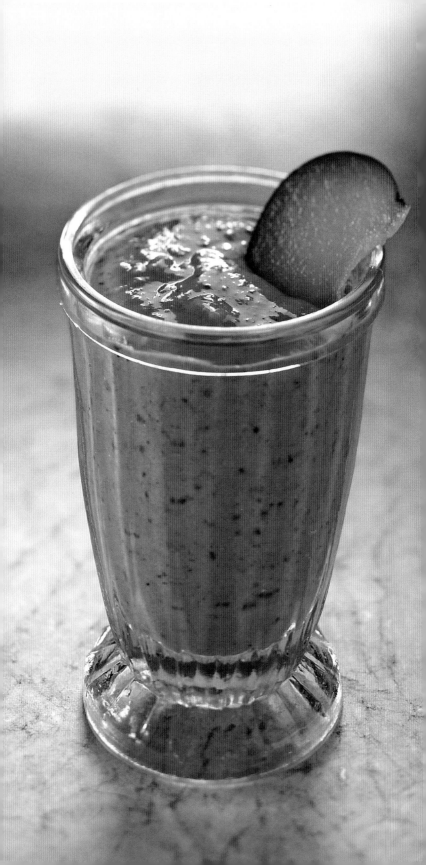

PHENOL-FILLED
PRUNE WHIP SMOOTHIE

Prunes are the dried form of plums, and both are high in phenols, which have long been touted for their antioxidant function. Phenols have been shown to inhibit oxygen-based damage to fats, including the fats that comprise a substantial proportion of our brain cells. This smoothie combines both forms of this sweet fruit, and is complemented by vitamin E-rich sunflower seeds for texture. The result is a complex and satisfying drink.

> 1 container (8 ounces or 225 g) vanilla low-fat yogurt
> 1/2 cup (120 ml) silken tofu
> 3/4 cup (130 g) unsulfured pitted prunes
> 1/2 cup (122 g) shelled sunflower seeds
> 1/4 cup (32 g) whey protein powder
> 2 fresh plums, pitted and sliced
> 4 green tea ice cubes
> 4 plum slices for garnish (optional)

■ Combine yogurt, tofu, prunes, sunflower seeds, whey protein powder, and plums in a blender or smoothie maker. Blend on high speed for 45 seconds or until mixture is puréed and smooth. Add ice cubes, and blend on high speed again until mixture is smooth. Serve immediately, garnished with plum slices, if desired.

■ **YIELD:** Four 1-cup (235-ml) servings

■ **NUTRITIONAL ANALYSIS:** Each 1-cup serving provides 274 calories; 10 g total fat; 2 g saturated fat; 13.5 g protein; 38 g carbohydrate; 4 g dietary fiber; 4 mg cholesterol.

■ **TIP:** Most dried fruit is rather soft, but if you find that your prunes—or any dried fruits—have hardened, it is best to rehydrate them before blending in a smoothie. The easiest way is to cover the fruit with boiling water or fruit juice for 10 to 20 minutes, depending on the size of the fruit.

SUPERCHARGE NUTRIENTS:	% DAILY VALUE*
Vitamin A	711.6 IU (14%)
Vitamin B6	0.3 mg (14%)
Vitamin C	3.3 mg (5%)
Vitamin E	8.2 mg (41%)
Magnesium	51.4 mg (13%)
Manganese	0.5 mg (24%)
Selenium	15.0 mcg (21%)
Zinc	1.4 mg (9%)

* Percent Daily Values are based on a 2,000 calorie diet. Your daily values may be higher or lower depending on your caloric needs.

BLADDER BUDDY
CREAMY ORANGE CRANBERRY SMOOTHIE

It is not an old wives' tale; cranberries do combat infections in the urinary tract, especially bladder infections; they also lower "bad" cholesterol.

3 navel oranges

1 container (8 ounces or 225 g) peach nonfat yogurt

1/2 cup (120 ml) silken tofu

1/2 cup (120 ml) freshly squeezed orange juice, chilled

1 package (3 ounces or 85 g) cream cheese, cut into 1/2 -inch (1-cm) pieces

1/4 cup (85 g) honey

1/4 cup (32 g) whey protein powder

2 tablespoons (30 g) bee pollen

1/2 teaspoon (1 g) ground ginger

2/3 cup (75 g) cranberries, frozen

4 orange segments for garnish (optional)

▓ Peel oranges, then slice off white pith. Cut around sides of sections to release segments from remaining pith. Cut into 1/2-inch (1-cm) dice.

▓ Combine oranges, yogurt, tofu, orange juice, cream cheese, honey, whey protein powder, bee pollen, and ginger in a blender or smoothie maker. Blend on high speed for 45 seconds or until mixture is puréed and smooth. Add cranberries, and blend on high speed again until mixture is smooth. Serve immediately, garnished with orange segments, if desired.

▓ **YIELD:** Four 1-cup (235-ml) servings

▓ **NUTRITIONAL ANALYSIS:** Each 1-cup serving provides 305 calories; 9 g total fat; 5 g saturated fat; 15 g protein; 45 g carbohydrate; 5 g dietary fiber; 43 mg cholesterol.

▓ **TIP:** Cranberries come to market in the fall. Buy a few extra bags and freeze the berries for smoothies and other dishes in other seasons.

SUPERCHARGE NUTRIENTS:	% DAILY VALUE*
Vitamin A	626.1 IU (13%)
Vitamin B6	0.2 mg (8%)
Vitamin C	79.1 mg (132%)
Vitamin E	1.2 mg (6%)
Magnesium	37.0 mg (9%)
Manganese	0.2 mg (9%)
Selenium	3.0 mcg (4%)
Zinc	1.2 mg (8%)

* Percent Daily Values are based on a 2,000 calorie diet. Your daily values may be higher or lower depending on your caloric needs.

BROMELAIN-BOASTING CITRUS PINEAPPLE SMOOTHIE

If you have problems with the innate acidity of citrus fruits causing tummy upset, then this is the smoothie for you! Pineapple contains bromelain, an enzyme that aids in digestion and reduces inflammation. All of these tropical fruits are also excellent sources of vitamin C, a nutrient that must be eaten regularly to keep your immune system primed.

2 navel oranges
1 red or pink grapefruit
1 cup (235 ml) silken tofu
1/4 cup (80 g) fruit-only orange marmalade
1/4 cup (32 g) whey protein powder
2 tablespoons (30 g) bee pollen
2 cups (330 g) pineapple cubes, frozen
4 pineapple spears for garnish (optional)

■ Peel oranges and grapefruit, then slice off white pith. Cut around sides of sections to release segments from remaining pith. Cut into 1/2-inch (1-cm) dice.

■ Combine oranges, grapefruit, tofu, orange marmalade, whey protein powder, and bee pollen in a blender or smoothie maker. Blend on high speed for 45 seconds or until mixture is puréed and smooth. Add pineapple, and blend on high speed again until mixture is smooth. Serve immediately, garnished with pineapple spears, if desired.

■ **YIELD:** Four 1-cup (235-ml) servings

■ **NUTRITIONAL ANALYSIS:** Each 1-cup serving provides 203 calories; 2 g total fat; 1 g saturated fat; 11 g protein; 40 g carbohydrate; 4 g dietary fiber; 18 mg cholesterol.

■ **TIP:** The red or pink grapefruit in this recipe not only adds phytonutrients, it also adds gives the smoothie a luscious pale pink color. If you are using a yellow grapefruit, you can compensate with 2 tablespoons (30 ml) of cranberry juice or pomegranate juice.

SUPERCHARGE NUTRIENTS:	% DAILY VALUE*
Vitamin A	339.8 IU (7%)
Vitamin B6	0.2 mg (9%)
Vitamin C	90.4 mg (151%)
Vitamin E	1.0 mg (5%)
Magnesium	34.1 mg (9%)
Manganese	0.9 mg (47%)
Selenium	1.4 mcg (2%)
Zinc	0.7 mg (5%)

Percent Daily Values are based on a 2,000 calorie diet. Your daily values may be higher or lower depending on your caloric needs.

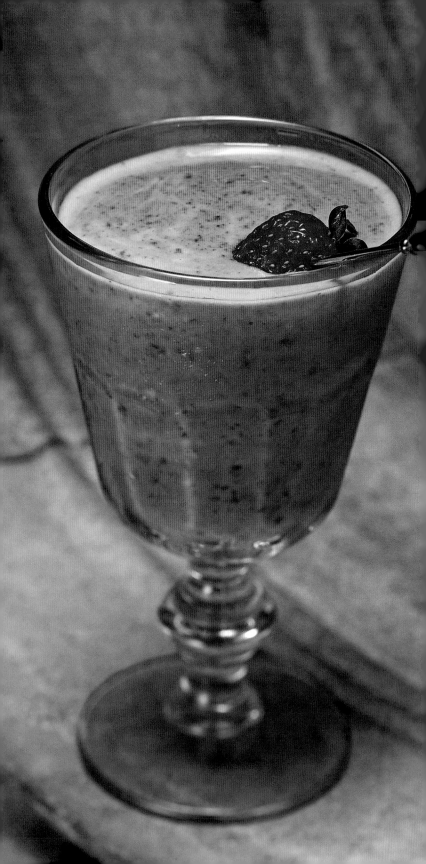

SUBLIMELY STRAWBERRY
C-LOADED SMOOTHIE

If you prefer smoothies with one dominant flavor rather than a blend of tastes, this is the recipe for you. Strawberries are not only a superb source of vitamin C, but they also contain a high amount of anthocyanin pigments, which give strawberries their rich red color and help to protect cell structures against oxidative damage.

> 1 container (8 ounces or 225 g) strawberry low-fat yogurt
> 3/4 cup (175 ml) plain soy milk
> 1/2 cup (120 ml) silken tofu
> 1/4 cup (32 g) whey protein powder
> 1/4 cup (80 g) fruit-only strawberry preserves
> 2 cups (290 g) strawberries, frozen
> 4 whole strawberries or strawberry fans for garnish (optional)

▒ Combine yogurt, soy milk, tofu, whey protein powder, and preserves in a blender or smoothie maker. Blend on high speed for 20 seconds or until mixture is puréed and smooth. Add strawberries, and blend on high speed again until mixture is smooth. Serve immediately, garnished with a strawberry fan, if desired.

▒ **YIELD:** Four 1-cup (235-ml) servings

▒ **NUTRITIONAL ANALYSIS:** Each 1-cup serving provides 205 calories; 2 g total fat; 1 g saturated fat; 11 g protein; 37 g carbohydrate; 2 g dietary fiber; 20 mg cholesterol.

▒ **TIP:** The strawberry season can be very short in parts of the world. Consider freezing berries to ensure that you have an ample supply throughout the year. First, hull and rinse the strawberries, pat dry with paper towels, and then freeze them on a baking sheet (small berries can be frozen whole; larger berries should be sliced). Once frozen, transfer the strawberries to a heavy resealable plastic bag and store in the freezer.

SUPERCHARGE NUTRIENTS:	% DAILY VALUE*
Vitamin A	161.8 IU (3%)
Vitamin B6	0.1 mg (4%)
Vitamin C	46.7 mg (78%)
Vitamin E	0.3 mg (2%)
Magnesium	35.8 mg (9%)
Manganese	0.4 mg (19%)
Selenium	2.8 mcg (4%)
Zinc	0.7 mg (4%)

* Percent Daily Values are based on a 2,000 calorie diet. Your daily values may be higher or lower depending on your caloric needs.

PERKY AND C-LICIOUS
WATERMELON STRAWBERRY SMOOTHIE

Tomatoes should not be your only source of valuable lycopene, an antioxi-dant shown to reduce the risk of heart disease. Thirst-quenching, low-calorie watermelon is another abundant source of this valued carotenoid. When watermelon is paired with two forms of strawberries, you get a vitamin C-filled smoothie with a vivid pink color and a delicious fruity flavor.

> 2 cups (300 g) seedless diced watermelon, chilled
> 1/2 cup (120 ml) silken tofu
> 1/4 cup (80 g) fruit-only strawberry preserves
> 2 tablespoons (30 g) bee pollen
> 1 tablespoon (15 ml) freshly squeezed lemon juice
> 1 1/2 cups (220 g) strawberries, frozen
> 1/2 cup (70 g) vanilla frozen yogurt
> 4 watermelon wedges or strawberry fans for garnish (optional)

■ Combine watermelon, tofu, strawberry preserves, bee pollen, and lemon juice in a blender or smoothie maker. Blend on high speed for 45 seconds or until mixture is puréed and smooth. Add strawberries and frozen yogurt, and blend on high speed again until mixture is smooth. Serve immediately, garnished with strawberry fans, if desired.

■ **YIELD:** Four 1-cup (235-ml) servings

■ **NUTRITIONAL ANALYSIS:** Each 1-cup serving provides 171 calories; 2 g total fat; 1 g saturated fat; 4 g protein; 37 g carbohydrate; 2 g dietary fiber; 2.5 mg cholesterol.

■ **TIP:** If you cannot find seedless watermelon—one of the great successes of genetic engineering—here is an easy way to remove the seeds. Dice the watermelon and place the flesh in a food processor fitted with a steel blade. After using on and off pulsing to chop, the seeds will be much easier to remove.

SUPERCHARGE NUTRIENTS:	% DAILY VALUE*
Vitamin A	358.2 IU (7%)
Vitamin B6	0.2 mg (9%)
Vitamin C	47.7 mg (79%)
Vitamin E	0.9 mg (5%)
Magnesium	26.8 mg (7%)
Manganese	0.3 mg (17%)
Selenium	2.7 mcg (4%)
Zinc	0.7 mg (4%)

* Percent Daily Values are based on a 2,000 calorie diet. Your daily values may be higher or lower depending on your caloric needs.

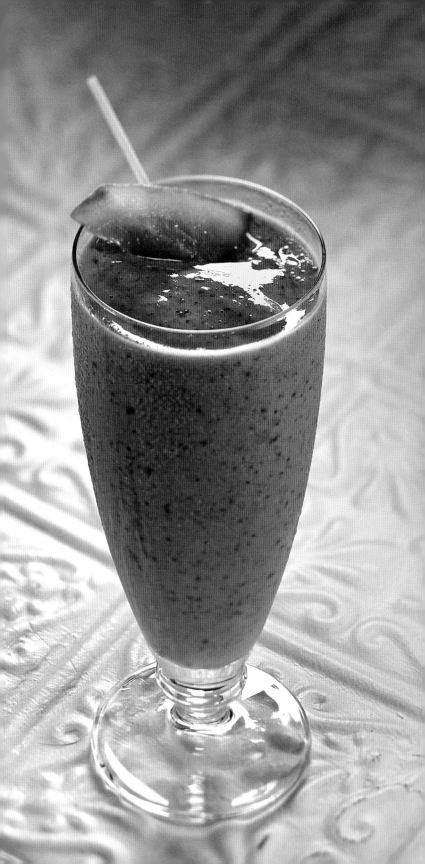

CELL-LICIOUS B6
WATERMELON BLUEBERRY SMOOTHIE

Vitamin B6 is needed for many metabolic reactions in the body, and low-calorie and refreshing watermelon is a good source of this nutrient, which also plays a role in new cell formation. When it is combined with antioxidant-powered blueberries, the resulting smoothie is light and delicious.

1 container (8 ounces or 225 g) blueberry nonfat yogurt
1 1/2 cups (225 g) diced seedless watermelon, chilled
1/4 cup (80 g) fruit-only blueberry preserves
1/4 cup (32 g) whey protein powder
2 tablespoons (30 g) bee pollen
2 cups (290 g) blueberries, frozen
4 watermelon spears for garnish (optional)

▓ Combine yogurt, watermelon, blueberry preserves, whey protein powder, and bee pollen in a blender or smoothie maker. Blend on high speed for 45 seconds or until mixture is puréed and smooth. Add blueberries, and blend on high speed again until mixture is smooth. Serve immediately, garnished with watermelon spears, if desired.

▓ **YIELD:** Four 1-cup (235-ml) servings

▓ **NUTRITIONAL ANALYSIS:** Each 1-cup serving provides 205 calories; 1 g total fat; 1 g saturated fat; 12 g protein; 39 g carbohydrate; 3 g dietary fiber; 20 mg cholesterol.

▓ **TIP:** There are now golden watermelon on the market in the same way that there are golden raspberries. However, the red color responsible for both traditional watermelon and raspberries contains a number of antioxidants, including lycopene, not found in the golden cousins.

SUPERCHARGE NUTRIENTS:	% DAILY VALUE*
Vitamin A . . . . 333.5 IU (7%)	
Vitamin B6 . . . . 0.1 mg (6%)	
Vitamin C . . . . 18.2 mg (30%)	
Vitamin E . . . . 1.4 mg (7%)	
Magnesium . . . . 32.1 mg (8%)	
Manganese . . . . 0.3 mg (16%)	
Selenium . . . . 2.5 mcg (4%)	
Zinc . . . . 1.0 mg (7%)	

* Percent Daily Values are based on a 2,000 calorie diet. Your daily values may be higher or lower depending on your caloric needs.

BETA-CAROTENE CONNECTION
SPICED WATERMELON MANGO SMOOTHIE

While watermelon, which is rich in vitamin B6, is refreshing to eat, it does not have the substance to star in a smoothie. That's where the mango, which boosts your immune system with its beta-carotene (which your body then converts to vitamin A), comes into play. Mango's more assertive texture and flavor blend wonderfully with the watermelon in this smoothie.

2 cups (300 g) diced seedless watermelon, chilled
1/2 cup (120 ml) mango nectar
1/3 cup (85 g) mango chutney
1/4 cup (32 g) whey protein powder
2 tablespoons (30 ml) flaxseed oil
1 1/2 cups (210 g) mango cubes, frozen
4 watermelon spears for garnish (optional)

▨ Combine watermelon, mango nectar, mango chutney, whey protein powder, and flaxseed oil in a blender or smoothie maker. Blend on high speed for 45 seconds or until mixture is puréed and smooth. Add mango cubes, and blend on high speed again until mixture is smooth. Serve immediately, garnished with watermelon spears, if desired.

▨ **YIELD:** Four 1-cup (235-ml) servings

▨ **NUTRITIONAL ANALYSIS:** Each 1-cup serving provides 178 calories; 7 g total fat; 1 g saturated fat; 7.5 g protein; 23.5 g carbohydrate; 2 g dietary fiber; 18 mg cholesterol.

▨ **TIP:** When dicing a juicy fruit like a mango or a pineapple, it is best to do it in a shallow bowl rather than on a cutting board. That way you can catch all of the resulting juices, and add them to the blender along with the fruit.

SUPERCHARGE NUTRIENTS:	% DAILY VALUE*
Vitamin A	3248.2 IU (65%)
Vitamin B6	0.1 mg (7%)
Vitamin C	32.2 mg (54%)
Vitamin E	2.1 mg (11%)
Magnesium	19.1 mg (5%)
Manganese	0.1 mg (3%)
Selenium	0.8 mcg (1%)
Zinc	0.1 mg (1%)

Percent Daily Values are based on a 2,000 calorie diet. Your daily values may be higher or lower depending on your caloric needs.

SAY C
STRAWBERRY MANGO BANANA SMOOTHIE

Aromatic sweet mangoes and luscious strawberries are both excellent sources of vitamin C, a powerful antioxidant the body uses to fight infection. In this blushing pink smoothie, they team up with creamy banana, which is high in the potassium your body needs to maintain normal blood pressure.

> 3/4 cup (175 ml) chilled mango nectar
> 1/2 cup (120 ml) silken tofu
> 1 cup (145 g) strawberries
> 1 cup (175 g) diced mango
> 1/4 cup (32 g) whey protein powder
> 2 tablespoons (30 g) bee pollen
> 1 cup (150 g) banana slices, frozen
> 8 mango spears for garnish (optional)

■ Combine mango nectar, tofu, strawberries, mango, whey protein powder, and bee pollen in a blender or smoothie maker. Blend on high speed for 45 seconds or until mixture is puréed and smooth. Add banana slices, and blend on high speed again until mixture is smooth. Serve immediately, garnished with mango spears, if desired.

■ **YIELD:** Four 1-cup (235-ml) servings

■ **NUTRITIONAL ANALYSIS:** Each 1-cup serving provides 184 calories; 2 g total fat; 1 g saturated fat; 10 g protein; 35.5 g carbohydrate; 3 g dietary fiber; 18 mg cholesterol.

■ **TIP:** You can buy a special strawberry huller that removes the fruit's green caps without grabbing the surrounding flesh, but you can also improvise one. A clean pair of tweezers or a binder clip serves the same function.

SUPERCHARGE NUTRIENTS:	% DAILY VALUE*
Vitamin A	1808.8 IU (36%)
Vitamin B6	0.5 mg (23%)
Vitamin C	48.7 mg (81%)
Vitamin E	1.3 mg (6%)
Magnesium	37.1 mg (9%)
Manganese	0.3 mg (13%)
Selenium	2.7 mcg (4%)
Zinc	0.7 mg (4%)

* Percent Daily Values are based on a 2,000 calorie diet. Your daily values may be higher or lower depending on your caloric needs.

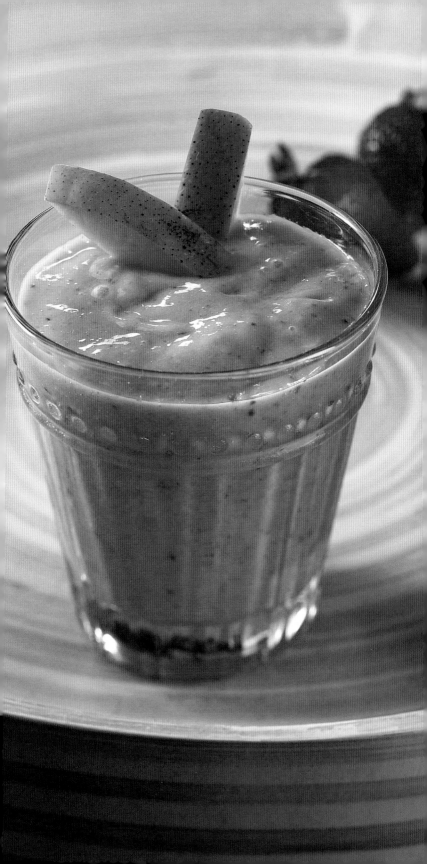

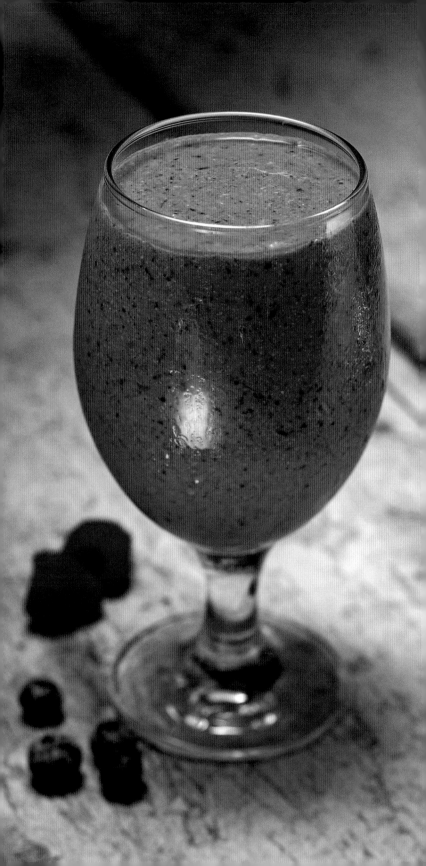

E-LICIOUS
PASTEL PUNCH SMOOTHIE

Vitamin E, a key nutrient found in crunchy sunflower seeds, neutralizes free radicals that might otherwise damage cell membranes and other fat-containing structures. This smoothie also features a healthy rainbow of sweet and delicious fruits.

1 cup (235 ml) purple grape juice
$1/2$ cup (120 ml) pomegranate juice or pomegranate-blueberry juice
$1/2$ cup (120 ml) silken tofu
$1/2$ cup (112 g) shelled sunflower seeds
1 container (4 ounces or 112 g) blueberry low-fat yogurt
1 medium banana, peeled and sliced
$1/2$ cup (75 g) blueberries, frozen
$1/2$ cup (75 g) raspberries, frozen
$1/2$ cup (70 g) vanilla frozen yogurt
16 fresh blueberries or raspberries threaded onto 4 skewers for garnish (optional)

▓ Combine grape juice, pomegranate juice, tofu, sunflower seeds, yogurt, and banana in a blender or smoothie maker. Blend on high speed for 45 seconds or until mixture is puréed and smooth. Add blueberries, raspberries, and frozen yogurt, and blend on high speed again until mixture is smooth. Serve immediately, garnished with berry skewers, if desired.

▓ **YIELD:** Four 1-cup (235-ml) servings

▓ **NUTRITIONAL ANALYSIS:** Each 1-cup serving provides 253 calories; 9 g total fat; 1.5 g saturated fat; 6 g protein; 39 g carbohydrate; 3 g dietary fiber; 3 mg cholesterol.

▓ **TIP:** Vanilla, found here in the frozen yogurt, enhances the sweet flavors of fruits. If you substitute another flavor of frozen yogurt for vanilla in a smoothie recipe, add a few drops of pure vanilla extract to the blend.

SUPERCHARGE NUTRIENTS:	% DAILY VALUE*
Vitamin A	89.0 IU (2%)
Vitamin B6	0.4 mg (19%)
Vitamin C	10.8 mg (18%)
Vitamin E	8.4 mg (42%)
Magnesium	46.7 mg (12%)
Manganese	0.9 mg (42%)
Selenium	14.7 mcg (21%)
Zinc	1.2 mg (8%)

* Percent Daily Values are based on a 2,000 calorie diet. Your daily values may be higher or lower depending on your caloric needs.

A-MAZING
SPICED PEACHY KEEN SMOOTHIE

Like all soy foods, tofu is a good source of manganese, iron, and selenium—all necessary trace minerals to boost your immunity. It adds a creamy texture to this smoothie based on a few forms of peaches, which are a good source of vitamin A and potassium for your immune system.

- 1 container (8 ounces or 225 g) peach low-fat yogurt
- 1/2 cup (120 ml) peach nectar
- 1/2 cup (120 ml) silken tofu
- 1/2 cup (120 ml) freshly squeezed orange juice
- 1/4 cup (80 g) fruit-only peach preserves
- 1/4 cup (32 g) whey protein powder
- 2 tablespoons (30 ml) flaxseed oil
- 2 tablespoons (30 g) bee pollen
- 1 teaspoon (2.5 g) apple pie spice
- 2 cups (340 g) peach slices, frozen
- 4 peach slices for garnish (optional)

▓ Combine yogurt, peach nectar, tofu, orange juice, peach preserves, whey protein powder, flaxseed oil, bee pollen, and apple pie spice in a blender or smoothie maker. Blend on high speed for 45 seconds or until mixture is puréed and smooth. Add peaches, and blend on high speed again until mixture is smooth. Serve immediately, garnished with peach slices, if desired.

▓ **YIELD:** Four 1-cup (235-ml) servings

▓ **NUTRITIONAL ANALYSIS:** Each 1-cup serving provides 266 calories; 8 g total fat; 1 g saturated fat; 13 g protein; 37 g carbohydrate; 2 g dietary fiber; 19.5 mg cholesterol.

▓ **TIP:** Apple pie spice is a blend of aromatic spices such as cinnamon, nutmeg, ginger, and ground cloves. Having it on hand is an easy and inexpensive way to add complex flavors to fruit desserts, but if you do not have it, use cinnamon or a combination of cinnamon and nutmeg.

SUPERCHARGE NUTRIENTS:	% DAILY VALUE*
Vitamin A	374.0 IU (7%)
Vitamin B6	0.1 mg (5 %)
Vitamin C	23.1 mg (39%)
Vitamin E	2.3 mg (11%)
Magnesium	32.7 mg (8%)
Manganese	0.1 mg (3%)
Selenium	2.3 mcg (3%)
Zinc	1.1 mg (7%)

* Percent Daily Values are based on a 2,000 calorie diet. Your daily values may be higher or lower depending on your caloric needs.

OPERATIC INSPIRATION
PEACH RASPBERRY SMOOTHIE

This smoothie is inspired by the dessert Peach Melba, named by famed chef Auguste Escoffier for opera singer Nellie Melba. Like the dessert, it combines peaches, which are a good source of beta-carotene, and antioxidant-rich bright, red raspberries.

1 container (8 ounces or 225 g) peach non-fat yogurt
1/2 cup (120 ml) silken tofu
1/4 cup (80 g) fruit-only peach preserves
1/4 cup (32 g) whey protein powder
1/4 cup (72 g) shelled sunflower seeds
2 tablespoons (30 g) bee pollen
1 cup (125 g) raspberries
2 cups (340 g) peach slices, frozen
4 peach slices for garnish (optional)

■ Combine yogurt, silken tofu, peach preserves, whey protein powder, sunflower seeds, bee pollen, and raspberries in a blender or smoothie maker. Blend on high speed for 45 seconds or until mixture is puréed and smooth. Add peach slices, and blend on high speed again until mixture is smooth. Serve immediately, garnished with peach slices, if desired.

■ **YIELD:** Four 1-cup (235-ml) servings

■ **NUTRITIONAL ANALYSIS:** Each 1-cup serving provides 253 calories; 6 g total fat; 1 g saturated fat; 15 g protein; 38 g carbohydrate; 5 g dietary fiber; 20 mg cholesterol.

■ **TIP:** Peaches and nectarines are similar in both flavor and nutritional content, so for smoothies they can be substituted for each other and it is always better to use a ripe nectarine rather than an unripe peach. Nectarines tend to be about half the size of a peach, so if a number is given rather than a cup or weight measurement, double the number.

SUPERCHARGE NUTRIENTS:	% DAILY VALUE*
Vitamin A	545.0 IU (11%)
Vitamin B6	0.2 mg (8%)
Vitamin C	20.2 mg (34%)
Vitamin E	5.4 mg (27%)
Magnesium	52.7 mg (13%)
Manganese	0.5 mg (24%)
Selenium	8.6 mcg (12%)
Zinc	1.7 mg (11%)

* Percent Daily Values are based on a 2,000 calorie diet. Your daily values may be higher or lower depending on your caloric needs.

VITAMIN A ODYSSEY
APRICOT PEACH SMOOTHIE

The bright orange color of apricots and peaches should serve as your clue that they are both good sources of beta-carotene, which helps protect your cells from free radicals, and lycopene, which may lower cholesterol and help prevent heart disease. These two fruits have complementary flavors as well as colors, as you will see when enjoying this frosty smoothie.

        1 cup (235 ml) chilled apricot nectar
        1/2 cup (120 ml) silken tofu
        1/2 cup (65 g) unsulfured dried apricots
        1 1/2 cups (255 g) peach slices, frozen
        1/2 cup (70 g) vanilla frozen yogurt
        4 peach wedges for garnish (optional)

■ Combine apricot nectar, tofu, and dried apricots in a blender or smoothie maker. Blend on high speed for 45 seconds or until mixture is puréed and smooth. Add peach slices and frozen yogurt, and blend on high speed again until mixture is smooth. Serve immediately, garnished with peach wedges, if desired.

■ **YIELD:** Four 1-cup (235-ml) servings

■ **NUTRITIONAL ANALYSIS:** Each 1-cup serving provides 180 calories; 1 g total fat; 0 g saturated fat; 3 g protein; 43 g carbohydrate; 4 g dietary fiber; 2.5 mg cholesterol.

■ **TIP:** Most commercial dried fruit has been sprayed with sulfur dioxide, a gas used for fumigation. The gas destroys much of the fruit's natural B vitamins, so make sure the dried fruit you buy is marked unsulfured.

SUPERCHARGE NUTRIENTS:	% DAILY VALUE*
Vitamin A	3628.5 IU (73%)
Vitamin B6	0.1 mg (5%)
Vitamin C	25.7 mg (43%)
Vitamin E	0.5 mg (3%)
Magnesium	27.4 mg (7%)
Manganese	0.2 mg (10%)
Selenium	2.7 mcg (4%)
Zinc	0.5 mg (3%)

* Percent Daily Values are based on a 2,000 calorie diet. Your daily values may be higher or lower depending on your caloric needs.

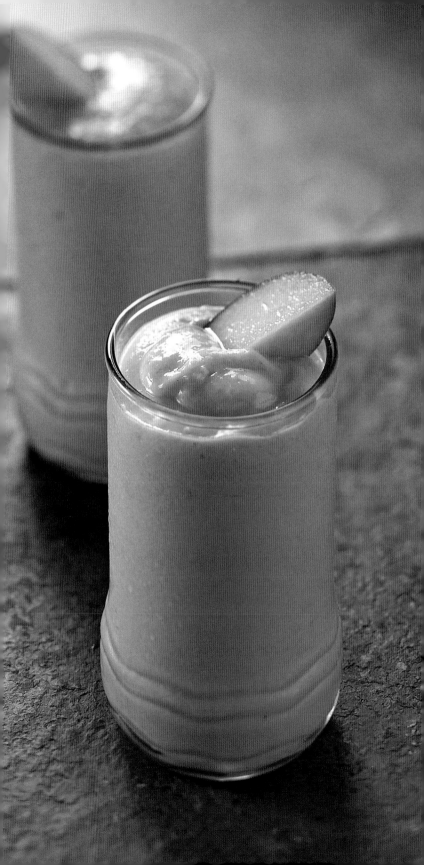

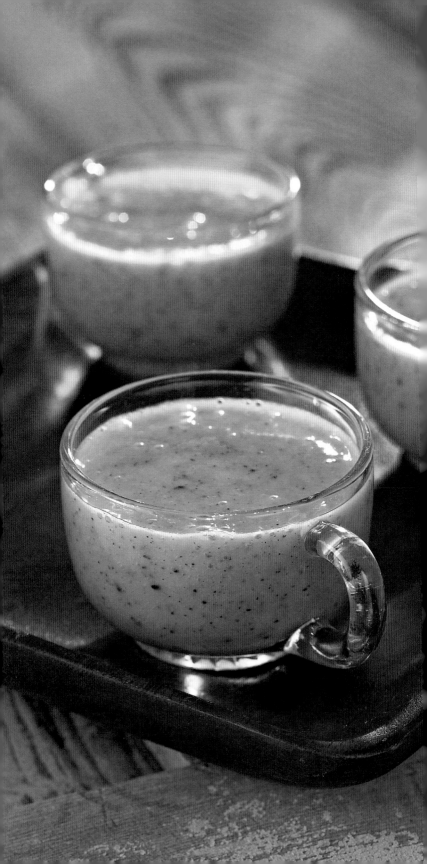

GREEN MACHINE
KIWI HONEYDEW SMOOTHIE

If you're looking for antioxidants, look no further than bright green kiwi-fruit, which contain a phytonutrient that helps to protect the DNA in human cells from oxygen-related damage. Moreover, they are a fabulous source of vitamin C. Here, the fruit's green color is enhanced by luscious, low-calorie honeydew melon, in a drink with a light, lemony taste.

- 1 container (8 ounces or 225 g) lemon low-fat yogurt
- 1/2 cup (120 ml) silken tofu
- 6 kiwifruit, peeled and diced
- 1 1/2 cups (255 g) diced honeydew melon
- 1/4 cup (32 g) whey protein powder
- 1/2 cup (75 g) lemon sorbet
- 4 kiwi slices for garnish (optional)

▓ Combine yogurt, tofu, kiwi, honeydew melon, and whey protein powder in a blender or smoothie maker. Blend on high speed for 45 seconds or until mixture is puréed and smooth. Add lemon sorbet, and blend on high speed again until mixture is smooth. Serve immediately, garnished with kiwi slices, if desired.

▓ **YIELD:** Four 1-cup (235-ml) servings

▓ **NUTRITIONAL ANALYSIS:** Each 1-cup serving provides 215 calories; 2 g total fat; 1 g saturated fat; 11 g protein; 41 g carbohydrate; 4 g dietary fiber; 22 mg cholesterol.

▓ **TIP:** If you object to seeing the kiwi fruit's black seeds in your smoothie, purée and strain the fruit to remove the seeds before continuing with the smoothie recipe. In contrast to fruits such as papaya, the seeds of a kiwi are totally edible.

SUPERCHARGE NUTRIENTS:	% DAILY VALUE*
Vitamin A	140.7 IU (3%)
Vitamin B6	0.2 mg (8%)
Vitamin C	123.2 mg (205%)
Vitamin E	1.4 mg (7%)
Magnesium	39.2 mg (10%)
Manganese	0.2 mg (9%)
Selenium	2.1 mcg (3%)
Zinc	0.6 mg (4%)

* Percent Daily Values are based on a 2,000 calorie diet. Your daily values may be higher or lower depending on your caloric needs.

DIVINE DNA
KIWI ORANGE SMOOTHIE

There is nothing as crucial to the body as your personal DNA, and the powerful antioxidants in kiwifruit are touted to protect DNA from free radical damage. When their high vitamin C level is added to that of oranges, you have a delicious smoothie ready to ward off any antigens coming your way.

> 2 navel oranges
> 1 container (8 ounces or 225 g) lemon low-fat yogurt
> 1/2 cup (120 ml) silken tofu
> 6 kiwifruit, peeled and diced
> 1/2 cup (75 g) shelled almonds, not skinned
> 1/4 cup (32 g) whey protein powder
> 2 tablespoons (30 g) bee pollen
> 3/4 cup (105 g) orange sorbet
> 4 slices kiwifruit for garnish (optional)

■ Peel oranges, then slice off white pith. Cut around sides of sections to release segments from remaining pith. Cut into 1/2-inch (1-cm) dice.

■ Combine oranges, yogurt, tofu, kiwifruit, almonds, whey protein powder, and bee pollen in a blender or smoothie maker. Blend on high speed for 45 seconds or until mixture is puréed and smooth. Add orange sorbet, and blend on high speed again until mixture is smooth. Serve immediately, garnished with kiwi slices, if desired.

■ **YIELD:** Four 1-cup (235-ml) servings

■ **NUTRITIONAL ANALYSIS:** Each 1-cup serving provides 326 calories; 9 g total fat; 1 g saturated fat; 16.5 g protein; 49 g carbohydrate; 7 g dietary fiber; 20 mg cholesterol.

■ **TIP:** Nuts, like the almonds in this recipe, are used as a thickening agent for foods like smoothies and sauces. Keep this in mind if cooking for someone on a gluten-free diet because traditional thickening ingredients like flour are not permitted.

SUPERCHARGE NUTRIENTS:	% DAILY VALUE*
Vitamin A	452.4 IU (9%)
Vitamin B6	0.2 mg (9%)
Vitamin C	168.9 mg (282%)
Vitamin E	2.8 mg (14%)
Magnesium	91.6 mg (23%)
Manganese	0.5 mg (26%)
Selenium	2.9 mcg (4%)
Zinc	1.7 mg (23%)

Percent Daily Values are based on a 2,000 calorie diet. Your daily values may be higher or lower depending on your caloric needs.

C IS FOR COLLAGEN
KIWI PINEAPPLE SMOOTHIE

Both bright green kiwifruit and vivid yellow pineapple are good sources of infection-fighting vitamin C, touted for being an excellent nutrient to keep your body in good shape as you age. Vitamin C is also involved in the production of collagen, which is found in connective tissue, cartilage, bone matrix, tooth dentin, skin, and tendons.

1 cup (235 ml) plain soy milk
1/2 cup (120 ml) pineapple juice
6 kiwifruit, peeled and diced
1/4 cup (32 g) whey protein powder
2 tablespoons (30 ml) flaxseed oil
2 cups (330 g) pineapple cubes, frozen
1/2 cup (70 g) vanilla frozen yogurt
4 slices kiwifruit for garnish (optional)

▓ Combine soy milk, pineapple juice, kiwifruit, whey protein powder, and flaxseed oil in a blender or smoothie maker. Blend on high speed for 45 seconds or until mixture is puréed and smooth. Add pineapple cubes and frozen yogurt, and blend on high speed again until mixture is smooth. Serve immediately, garnished with kiwifruit slices, if desired.

▓ **YIELD:** Four 1-cup (235-ml) servings

▓ **NUTRITIONAL ANALYSIS:** Each 1-cup serving provides 264 calories; 9 g total fat; 1 g saturated fat; 11 g protein; 38 g carbohydrate; 5 g dietary fiber; 21 mg cholesterol.

▓ **TIP:** If you do not want to lose much of a pineapple's juicy flesh by cutting off the skin too deeply, you are frequently left with woody "eyes" dotting the yellow fruit. An easy way to rid the pineapple of these "eyes" is with the tip of a paring knife; if you use it in a circular fashion they come out easily.

SUPERCHARGE NUTRIENTS:	% DAILY VALUE*
Vitamin A	395.2 IU (8%)
Vitamin B6	0.2 mg (9%)
Vitamin C	136.7 mg (228%)
Vitamin E	2.5 mg (13%)
Magnesium	46.5 mg (12%)
Manganese	1.4 mg (69%)
Selenium	0.4 mcg (1%)
Zinc	0.4 mg (3%)

* Percent Daily Values are based on a 2,000 calorie diet. Your daily values may be higher or lower depending on your caloric needs.

PRIMING THE PUMP
CITRUS GREEN TEA SMOOTHIE

Green tea contains an antigen that does not fully activate the body's T-cells, but it does keep them in a state of readiness so that when bacteria arrive, the cells are ready to fight. Another benefit to this smoothie is the high amount of vitamin C in the citrus fruits, which pumps up the antioxidant level.

> 4 navel oranges
> 2 large red or pink grapefruit
> 1/4 cup (80 g) fruit-only orange marmalade
> 2 tablespoons (30 ml) flaxseed oil
> 2 tablespoons (30 g) bee pollen
> 8 green tea ice cubes
> 4 orange slices or peels for garnish (optional)

■ Peel oranges and grapefruit, and slice off white pith. Cut around sides of sections to release segments from remaining pith. Cut into 1/2-inch (1-cm) dice.

■ Combine orange and grapefruit sections, orange marmalade, flaxseed oil, and bee pollen in a blender or smoothie maker. Blend on high speed for 45 seconds or until mixture is puréed and smooth. Add ice cubes, and blend on high speed again until mixture is smooth. Serve immediately, garnished with orange slices, if desired.

■ **YIELD:** Four 1-cup (235-ml) servings

■ **NUTRITIONAL ANALYSIS:** Each 1-cup serving provides 237 calories; 7 g total fat; 1 g saturated fat; 4 g protein; 43.5 g carbohydrate; 2 g dietary fiber; 0 mg cholesterol.

■ **TIP:** While it might seem useful to peel citrus fruits early in the day to make a smoothie at lunchtime, resist the temptation. Citrus fruit begins to lose its vitamin-C content almost as soon as it is exposed to oxygen, so the nutrient value drops if the fruit sits for longer than a few minutes.

SUPERCHARGE NUTRIENTS:	% DAILY VALUE*
Vitamin A	584.0 IU (12%)
Vitamin B6	0.2 mg (9%)
Vitamin C	130.7 mg (218%)
Vitamin E	2.0 mg (10%)
Magnesium	28.1 mg (7%)
Manganese	0.05 mg (3%)
Selenium	1.8 mcg (3%)
Zinc	0.6 mg (7%)

Percent Daily Values are based on a 2,000 calorie diet. Your daily values may be higher or lower depending on your caloric needs.

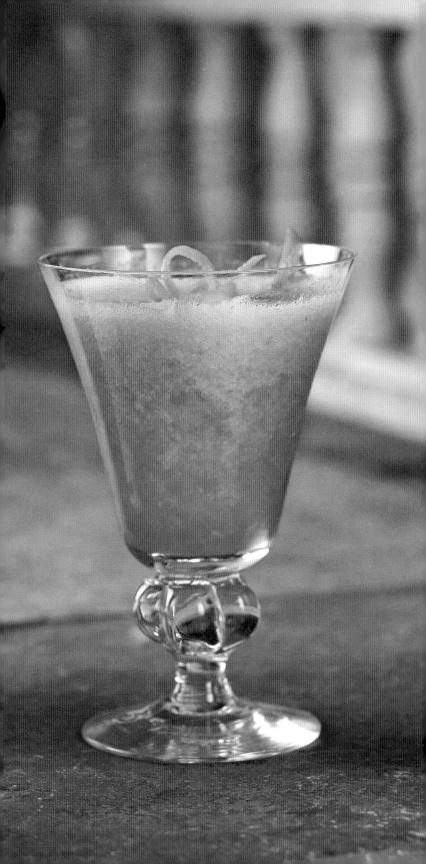

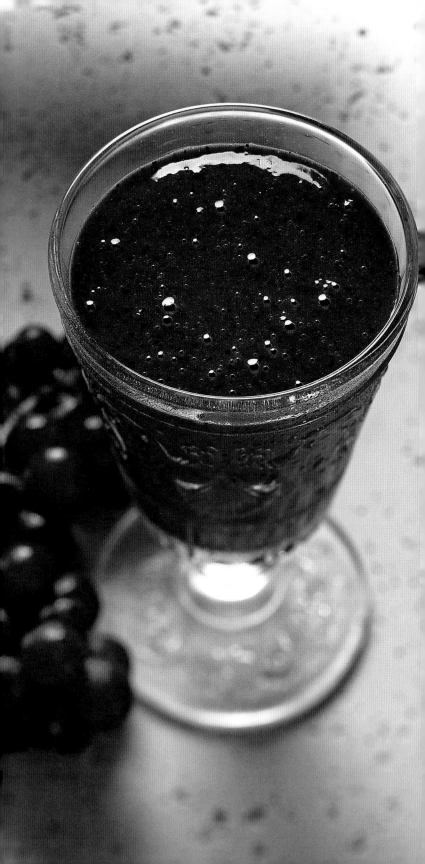

RAVES FOR RESVERATROL GRAPE BLUEBERRY SMOOTHIE

Flavonoids, which give red grapes and blueberries their vibrant colors, are phytonutrients that are extremely helpful to the body. Grapes, along with blueberries, peanuts, and red wine, contain resveratrol, an antioxidant that may help reduce the risk of heart disease.

1 cup (235 ml) chilled purple grape juice
1/2 cup (120 ml) silken tofu
1/4 cup (32 g) whey protein powder
2 tablespoons (40 g) fruit-only grape jelly
1 1/2 cups (220 g) blueberries
1 1/2 cups (240 g) red seedless grapes, frozen
12 red seedless grapes threaded onto 4 toothpicks for garnish (optional)

▓ Combine grape juice, tofu, whey protein powder, grape jelly, and blueberries in a blender or smoothie maker. Blend on high speed for 45 seconds or until mixture is puréed and smooth. Add grapes, and blend on high speed again until mixture is smooth. Serve immediately, garnished with grape skewers, if desired.

▓ **YIELD:** Four 1-cup (235-ml) servings

▓ **NUTRITIONAL ANALYSIS:** Each 1-cup serving provides 181 calories; 1 g total fat; 0 g saturated fat; 8 g protein; 37 g carbohydrate; 2 g dietary fiber; 18 mg cholesterol.

▓ **TIP:** Frozen grapes are nature's best ice cubes. Unlike most frozen fruits that lend their flavor to whatever drink they are chilling, the juice from frozen grapes remains in the skin. After the grapes have thawed and you've enjoyed a cool drink, eat the grapes to help satisfy your daily fruit requirements.

SUPERCHARGE NUTRIENTS:	% DAILY VALUE*
Vitamin A	120.7 IU (2%)
Vitamin B6	0.1 mg (7%)
Vitamin C	13.7 mg (23%)
Vitamin E	1.0 mg (5%)
Magnesium	20.6 mg (5%)
Manganese	0.5 mg (3%)
Selenium	2.3 mcg (3%)
Zinc	0.2 mg (1%)

* Percent Daily Values are based on a 2,000 calorie diet. Your daily values may be higher or lower depending on your caloric needs.

ANTIOXIDANT-ABUNDANT GRAPE KIWI SMOOTHIE

Not only are grapes a great source of immune-boosting manganese, but their skins contain resveratrol, a powerful antioxidant. So when you combine grapes with kiwifruit—a leader in vitamin-C content—your immune system gets double the boost.

> 1 cup (235 ml) chilled white grape juice
> 1/2 cup (120 ml) silken tofu
> 6 kiwifruit, peeled and diced
> 1/4 cup (32 g) whey protein powder
> 2 cups (320 g) green grapes, frozen
> 4 kiwi slices for garnish (optional)

■ Combine grape juice, tofu, kiwifruit, and whey protein powder in a blender or smoothie maker. Blend on high speed for 45 seconds or until mixture is puréed and smooth. Add grapes, and blend on high speed again until mixture is smooth. Serve immediately, garnished with kiwi slices, if desired.

■ **YIELD:** Four 1-cup (235-ml) servings

■ **NUTRITIONAL ANALYSIS:** Each 1-cup serving provides 208 calories; 2 g total fat; 0.5 g saturated fat; 9 g protein; 43 g carbohydrate; 5 g dietary fiber; 18 mg cholesterol.

■ **TIP:** When making a smoothie, having neat slices of kiwi is irrelevant, so here is an easy way to prepare them for blending: Cut each fruit in half and use a serrated grapefruit spoon to remove the pulp, leaving the brown skin behind. You will find this technique much faster than peeling the furry fruit.

SUPERCHARGE NUTRIENTS:	% DAILY VALUE*
Vitamin A	278.8 IU (6%)
Vitamin B6	0.1 mg (7%)
Vitamin C	94.2 mg (157%)
Vitamin E	1.8 mg (9%)
Magnesium	52.7 mg (13%)
Manganese	0.33 mg (17%)
Selenium	2.5 mcg (4%)
Zinc	0.2 mg (1%)

* Percent Daily Values are based on a 2,000 calorie diet. Your daily values may be higher or lower depending on your caloric needs.

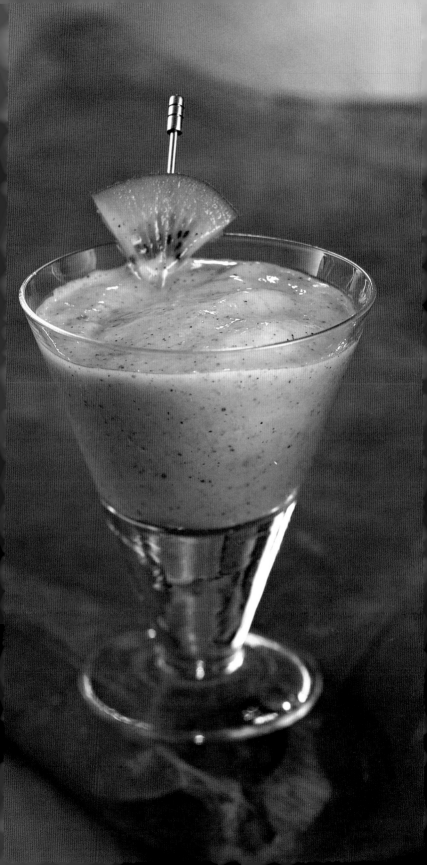

POLYPHENOL PLEASURES
PLUM GRAPE SMOOTHIE

The purple skin and flesh of plums is loaded with antioxidant polyphenols, and their flavor and color blend beautifully with red grapes and purple grape juice. Red grapes are an excellent source of resveratrol, which is posited to reduce the risk of heart disease and cancer.

> 1 cup (235 ml) chilled purple grape juice
> 1/2 cup (120 ml) silken tofu
> 2 tablespoons (40 g) fruit-only grape jelly
> 1/4 cup (32 g) whey protein powder
> 2 tablespoons (30 g) bee pollen
> 2 cups (450 g) diced plums
> 1 1/2 cups (240 g) red seedless grapes, frozen
> 4 plum wedges for garnish (optional)

■ Combine grape juice, tofu, grape jelly, whey protein powder, bee pollen, and plums in a blender or smoothie maker. Blend on high speed for 45 seconds or until mixture is puréed and smooth. Add grapes, and blend on high speed again until mixture is smooth. Serve immediately, garnished with plum wedges, if desired.

■ **YIELD:** Four 1-cup (235-ml) servings

■ **NUTRITIONAL ANALYSIS:** Each 1-cup serving provides 192 calories; 2 g total fat; 1 g saturated fat; 11 g protein; 35 g carbohydrate; 2 g dietary fiber; 18 mg cholesterol.

■ **TIP:** Plums are one species of fruit that vary greatly in both size and color. The "average size" plum is about 2 1/2-inches (6.5-cm) long. While this recipe calls for volume/weight measure, use this size as a general guide for plums and if you have small Italian prune plums, use 1 1/2 for each plum specified.

SUPERCHARGE NUTRIENTS:	% DAILY VALUE*
Vitamin A	321.0 IU (6%)
Vitamin B6	0.1 mg (7%)
Vitamin C	13.1 mg (22%)
Vitamin E	1.4 mg (7%)
Magnesium	26.7 mg (7%)
Manganese	0.3 mg (15%)
Selenium	0.1 mcg (0%)
Zinc	0.7 mg (4%)

* Percent Daily Values are based on a 2,000 calorie diet. Your daily values may be higher or lower depending on your caloric needs.

SPLENDID SAPONINS
GRAPE MANGO SMOOTHIE

Move over, red grapes: green grapes are a heart-healthy fruit, too. They contain flavonoid compounds including quercetin, which can reduce the risk of atherosclerosis. They also contain saponins, which may help to reduce the reabsorption of cholesterol. Blended with mango, which is high in both vitamin C and beta-carotene, the resulting smoothie will keep your immune system in tip-top shape.

- 1/2 cup (120 ml) chilled white grape juice
- 1/2 cup (120 ml) chilled mango nectar
- 1/2 cup (120 ml) silken tofu
- 1/4 cup (32 g) whey protein powder
- 2 tablespoons (30 g) bee pollen
- 1 1/2 cups (265 g) diced mango
- 1 1/2 cups (240 g) green seedless grapes, frozen
- 4 mango spears for garnish (optional)

▓ Combine grape juice, mango nectar, tofu, whey protein powder, bee pollen, and mango in a blender or smoothie maker. Blend on high speed for 45 seconds or until mixture is puréed and smooth. Add grapes, and blend on high speed again until mixture is smooth. Serve immediately, garnished with mango spears, if desired.

▓ **YIELD:** Four 1-cup (235-ml) servings

▓ **NUTRITIONAL ANALYSIS:** Each 1-cup serving provides 172 calories; 2 g total fat; 1 g saturated fat; 11 g protein; 31 g carbohydrate; 2 g dietary fiber; 18 mg cholesterol.

▓ **TIP:** It is now very easy to find seedless grapes on the market; the genetic engineering of these species to omit the seeds was a great advancement of science. If you mistakenly buy grapes with seeds, it is important to remove them. They will give the smoothie a bitter under-state and unappealing texture.

SUPERCHARGE NUTRIENTS:	% DAILY VALUE*
Vitamin A	2454.5 IU (49%)
Vitamin B6	0.2 mg (9%)
Vitamin C	39.1 mg (65%)
Vitamin E	1.6 mg (8%)
Magnesium	25.1 mg (6%)
Manganese	0.1 mg (4%)
Selenium	0.4 mcg (1%)
Zinc	0.6 mg (4%)

* Percent Daily Values are based on a 2,000 calorie diet. Your daily values may be higher or lower depending on your caloric needs.

ENZYME-ACTIVATING
MANGO RASPBERRY SMOOTHIE

Raspberries are a superb source of manganese, an important mineral that activates the enzymes responsible for using other key nutrients to boost your immune system. Raspberries' succulent flavor is a great match for the aromatic richness of mango, which is high in antioxidant vitamin C.

1 container (8 ounces or 225 g) raspberry low-fat yogurt

1/2 cup (120 ml) chilled mango nectar

3/4 cup (95 g) raspberries

1/4 cup (32 g) whey protein powder

2 tablespoons (30 g) bee pollen

1 1/2 cups (250 g) mango slices, frozen

1/2 cup (70 g) raspberry sorbet

4 peach or mango slices for garnish (optional)

■ Combine yogurt, mango nectar, raspberries, whey protein powder, and bee pollen in a blender or smoothie maker. Blend on high speed for 45 seconds or until mixture is puréed and smooth. Add mango slices and sorbet, and blend on high speed again until mixture is smooth. Serve immediately, garnished with peach or mango slices, if desired.

■ **YIELD:** Four 1-cup (235-ml) servings

■ **NUTRITIONAL ANALYSIS:** Each 1-cup serving provides 199 calories; 2 g total fat; 1 g saturated fat; 11 g protein; 37 g carbohydrate; 3 g dietary fiber; 22 mg cholesterol.

■ **TIP:** Mangoes are aromatic, sweet, and luscious when ripe and unbelievably bitter when unripe, and it can take up to a week to ripen a hard mango. While the nutritional profile will be altered somewhat, you can substitute ripe papaya for unripe mango in any recipe.

SUPERCHARGE NUTRIENTS:	% DAILY VALUE*
Vitamin A	1557.7 IU (51%)
Vitamin B6	0.2 mg (8%)
Vitamin C	32.9 mg (55%)
Vitamin E	1.4 mg (7%)
Magnesium	18.3 mg (5%)
Manganese	0.3 mg (12%)
Selenium	0.5 mcg (1%)
Zinc	0.5 mg (4%)

* Percent Daily Values are based on a 2,000 calorie diet. Your daily values may be higher or lower depending on your caloric needs.

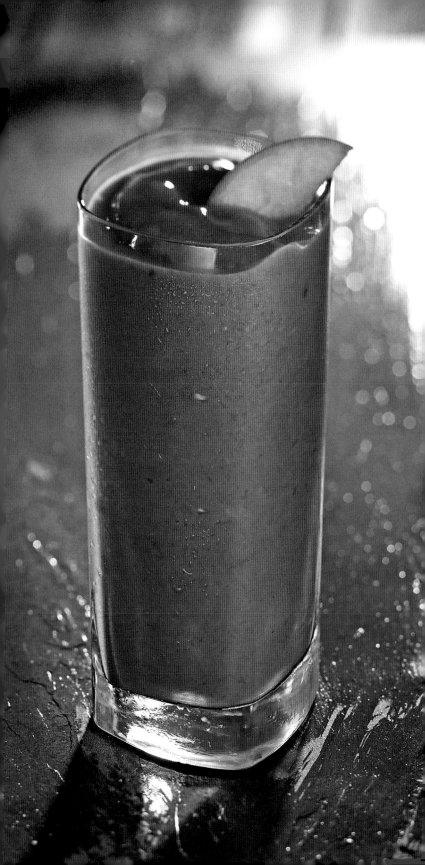

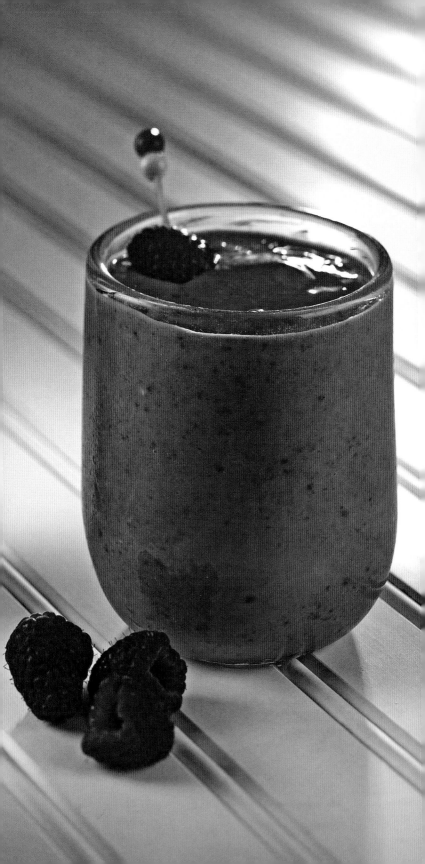

ELLAGIC EXCITEMENT
RASPBERRY BANANA SMOOTHIE

Many health food stores sell ellagic acid, which has antiviral, antibacterial, and anticarcinogenic properties, but raspberries are your naturally delicious, go-to food source for this powerful antioxidant phytonutrient. In addition, the flavonoids that give raspberries their red color are an immunity booster, and raspberries and bananas are both good sources of fiber.

- 1 container (8 ounces or 225 g) raspberry low-fat yogurt
- 1/2 cup (120 ml) silken tofu
- 1/4 cup (80 g) fruit-only raspberry preserves
- 1/4 cup (32 g) whey protein powder
- 2 tablespoons (30 g) bee pollen
- 2 cups (300 g) sliced banana
- 1 1/2 cups (190 g) raspberries, frozen
- 12 raspberries threaded onto 4 toothpicks for garnish (optional)

■ Combine yogurt, tofu, raspberry preserves, whey protein powder, bee pollen, and banana in a blender or smoothie maker. Blend on high speed for 45 seconds or until mixture is puréed and smooth. Add raspberries, and blend on high speed again until mixture is smooth. Serve immediately, garnished with raspberry skewers, if desired.

■ **YIELD:** Four 1-cup (235-ml) servings

■ **NUTRITIONAL ANALYSIS:** Each 1-cup serving provides 300 calories; 2 g total fat; 1 g saturated fat; 13 g protein; 61 g carbohydrate; 5 g dietary fiber; 22 mg cholesterol.

■ **TIP:** The best way to rinse delicate berries like raspberries and blackberries is to place them in a bowl of cold water, swirl them around gently, and remove them with a slotted spoon. Placing berries in a strainer under cold running water can bruise them.

SUPERCHARGE NUTRIENTS:	% DAILY VALUE*
Vitamin A	168.5 IU (3%)
Vitamin B6	0.8 mg (38%)
Vitamin C	28.3 mg (47%)
Vitamin E	1.1 mg (6%)
Magnesium	53.5 mg (13%)
Manganese	0.7 mg (35%)
Selenium	3.6 mcg (5%)
Zinc	0.9 mg (6%)

Percent Daily Values are based on a 2,000 calorie diet. Your daily values may be higher or lower depending on your caloric needs.

LOVE THAT LYCOPENE
APRICOT ALMOND SMOOTHIE

It is not just tomatoes that can tout the virtues of the powerful antioxidant lycopene in your diet; vitamin A-rich apricots are also an excellent source. In this smoothie, the vibrant flavor and vivid orange color from the fruit is juxtaposed with that of delicate almonds, rich in both vitamin E and manganese.

- 1 container (8 ounces or 225 g) peach nonfat yogurt
- 1/2 cup (120 ml) silken tofu
- 1/2 cup (120 ml) apricot nectar
- 3/4 cup (135 g) dried apricots, diced
- 1/2 cup (75 g) shelled almonds, not skinned
- 1/4 cup (32 g) whey protein powder
- 2 tablespoons (30 g) bee pollen
- 1/2 teaspoon (2.5 ml) pure almond extract
- 2 cups (330 g) apricot slices, frozen
- 4 apricot slices for garnish (optional)

▓ Combine yogurt, tofu, apricot nectar, dried apricots, almonds, whey protein powder, bee pollen, and almond extract in a blender or smoothie maker. Blend on high speed for 45 seconds or until mixture is puréed and smooth. Add apricot slices, and blend on high speed again until mixture is smooth. Serve immediately, garnished with apricot slices, if desired.

▓ **YIELD:** Four 1-cup (235-ml) servings

▓ **NUTRITIONAL ANALYSIS:** Each 1-cup serving provides 355 calories; 9 g total fat; 1 g saturated fat; 18 g protein; 57 g carbohydrate; 8 g dietary fiber; 20 mg cholesterol.

▓ **TIP:** Fresh, ripe apricots are also a good source of dietary fiber because there is no reason to peel the thin skin. If you want to freeze apricots for smoothies or cakes in the winter months, it is best to cut them into slices or cubes no larger than 1-inch.

SUPERCHARGE NUTRIENTS:	% DAILY VALUE*
Vitamin A	6114.6 IU (122%)
Vitamin B6	0.2 mg (12%)
Vitamin C	30.1 mg (50%)
Vitamin E	2.1 mg (10%)
Magnesium	85.2 mg (21%)
Manganese	1.0 mg (50%)
Selenium	3.9 mcg (6%)
Zinc	1.8 mg (21%)

* Percent Daily Values are based on a 2,000 calorie diet. Your daily values may be higher or lower depending on your caloric needs.

INFLAMMATION-FIGHTING
APRICOT BLACKBERRY SMOOTHIE

The vivid flavors of apricots and blackberries join together wonderfully in this luscious, lavender-colored smoothie. Blackberries are an excellent source of flavonoids, which reduce inflammation in the body and are also antiviral, and apricots add their own antioxidant punch.

1 cup (235 ml) apricot nectar
$^1/_2$ cup (120 ml) silken tofu
$^1/_2$ cup (135 g) dried apricots, diced
2 ripe apricots, stoned and diced
$^1/_4$ cup (32 g) whey protein powder
2 tablespoons (30 g) bee pollen
2 tablespoons (30 ml) flaxseed oil
2 cups (290 g) blackberries, frozen
$^1/_2$ cup (70 g) lemon sorbet
4 apricot wedges for garnish (optional)

▓ Combine apricot nectar, tofu, dried apricots, fresh apricots, whey protein powder, bee pollen, and flaxseed oil in a blender or smoothie maker. Blend on high speed for 45 seconds or until mixture is puréed and smooth. Add blackberries and lemon sorbet, and blend on high speed again until mixture is smooth. Serve immediately, garnished with apricot wedges, if desired.

▓ **YIELD:** Four 1-cup (235-ml) servings

▓ **NUTRITIONAL ANALYSIS:** Each 1-cup serving provides 307 calories; 8 g total fat; 1 g saturated fat; 13 g protein; 51 g carbohydrate; 8 g dietary fiber; 18 mg cholesterol.

▓ **TIP:** People suffering from intestinal distress, especially diverticulitis, are frequently told to eliminate nuts and seeds from their diets. To avoid the pronounced seeds found berries like blackberries and raspberries, purée them in a food processor and then strain off the seeds. Do not purée them in a blender, however, as the seeds will be crushed too small to strain.

SUPERCHARGE NUTRIENTS:	% DAILY VALUE*
Vitamin A	3912.1 IU (78%)
Vitamin B6	0.1 mg (6%)
Vitamin C	37.3 mg (62%)
Vitamin E	2.6 mg (13%)
Magnesium	40.7 mg (10%)
Manganese	0.6 mg (29%)
Selenium	1.2 mcg (2%)
Zinc	1.1 mg (7%)

* Percent Daily Values are based on a 2,000 calorie diet. Your daily values may be higher or lower depending on your caloric needs.

BRIGHT EYES
ABSOLUTELY APRICOT SMOOTHIE

The beta-carotene that your body converts to vitamin A is important for regulating your immune system, as it helps the skin and mucous membranes function as a barrier to bacteria. The vitamin is also crucial for maintaining good vision because it promotes healthy surface linings in the eyes. Apricots are an excellent source of vitamin A, and when three different forms of this vivid orange fruit are combined into one smoothie, their succulent flavor is magnified.

> 1 cup (235 ml) chilled apricot nectar
> 1/2 cup (120 ml) silken tofu
> 1 cup (175 g) firmly packed dried apricot halves, diced
> 1/4 cup (32 g) whey protein powder
> 1 1/2 cups (250 g) apricot slices, frozen
> 1/2 cup (70 g) vanilla frozen yogurt
> 4 apricot slices for garnish (optional)

■ Combine apricot nectar, tofu, dried apricots, and whey protein powder in a blender or smoothie maker. Blend on high speed for 45 seconds or until mixture is puréed and smooth. Add frozen apricot slices and frozen yogurt, and blend on high speed again until mixture is smooth. Serve immediately, garnished with apricot slices, if desired.

■ **YIELD:** Four 1-cup (235-ml) servings

■ **NUTRITIONAL ANALYSIS:** Each 1-cup serving provides 256 calories; 2 g total fat; 1 g saturated fat; 11 g protein; 54 g carbohydrate; 6 g dietary fiber; 21 mg cholesterol.

■ **TIP:** The skin on apricots is so thin that peeling them is unnecessary. But you should rinse them well before removing the stone; the soft skin can harbor lingering grit from harvest and shipping.

SUPERCHARGE NUTRIENTS:	% DAILY VALUE*
Vitamin A	6678.9 IU (134%)
Vitamin B6	0.2 mg (8%)
Vitamin C	11.6 mg (19%)
Vitamin E	0.9 mg (5%)
Magnesium	39.2 mg (10%)
Manganese	0.3 mg (14%)
Selenium	3.0 mcg (4%)
Zinc	0.7 mg (5%)

* Percent Daily Values are based on a 2,000 calorie diet. Your daily values may be higher or lower depending on your caloric needs.

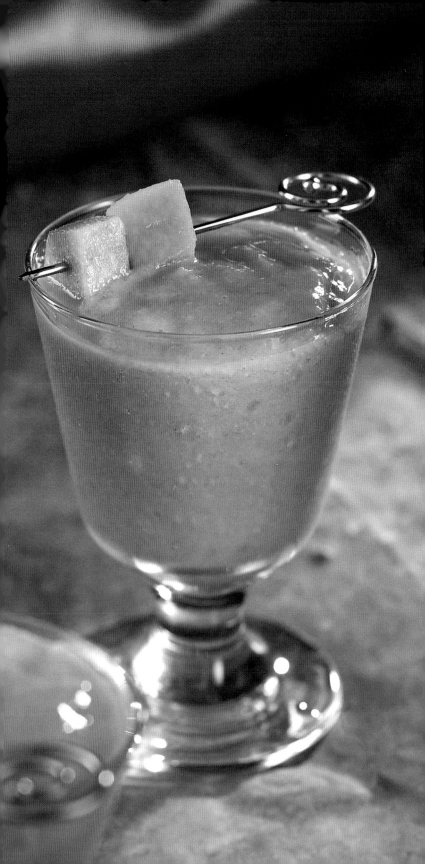

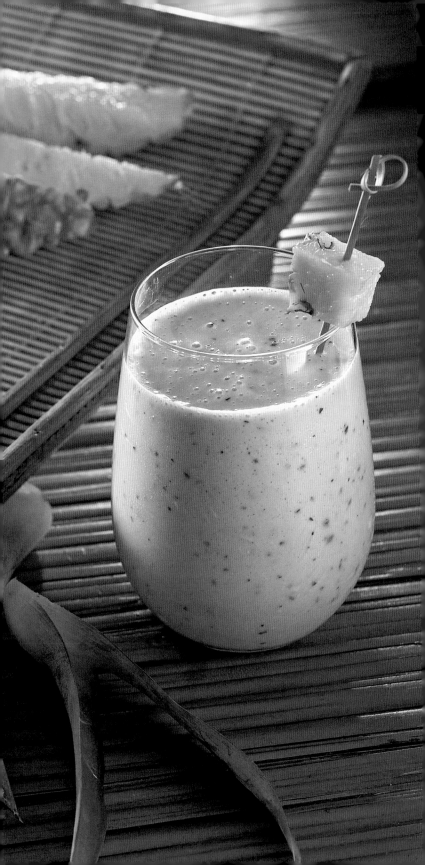

PHILLED WITH PHENOLS
PINEAPPLE PLUM SMOOTHIE

Plums and their dried-form, prunes, are high in phytonutrients, classified as phenols, and provide antioxidant muscle for your body. In addition, they contain iron, which is more readily absorbed when taken with vitamin C, a nutrient found in pinapple.

> 1 container (8 ounces or 225 g) plain low-fat yogurt
> 1/2 cup (120 ml) silken tofu
> 1 1/2 cups (235 g) diced pineapple
> 1/4 cup (32 g) whey protein powder
> 2 tablespoons (30 g) bee pollen
> 1 cup (165 g) diced plums, frozen
> 4 pineapple spears for garnish (optional)

▨ Combine yogurt, tofu, pineapple, whey protein powder, and bee pollen in a blender or smoothie maker. Blend on high speed for 45 seconds or until mixture is puréed and smooth. Add plums, and blend on high speed again until mixture is smooth. Serve immediately, garnished with pineapple spears, if desired.

▨ **YIELD:** Four 1-cup (235-ml) servings

▨ **NUTRITIONAL ANALYSIS:** Each 1-cup serving provides 146 calories; 2 g total fat; 1 g saturated fat; 12 g protein; 22 g carbohydrate; 2 g dietary fiber; 19.5 mg cholesterol.

▨ **TIP:** Here is the best way to remove the skin from a pineapple: Cut off the two ends and stand the fruit firmly on the counter. Use a serrated knife to remove the skin, digging out any remaining eyes with the tip of the knife. Slice the pineapple into quarters, discard the woody core, and cut into whatever size pieces you prefer.

SUPERCHARGE NUTRIENTS:	% DAILY VALUE*
Vitamin A	166.1 IU (3%)
Vitamin B6	0.2 mg (8%)
Vitamin C	17.1 mg (29%)
Vitamin E	0.9 mg (5%)
Magnesium	30.1 mg (8%)
Manganese	1.0 mg (52%)
Selenium	4.2 mcg (6%)
Zinc	1.0 mg (7%)

* Percent Daily Values are based on a 2,000 calorie diet. Your daily values may be higher or lower depending on your caloric needs.

MAKE MINE MANGANESE
CREAMY PINEAPPLE STRAWBERRY SMOOTHIE

The cream cheese makes this smoothie rather indulgent, but it does contain many nutrients necessary for your immune system. Pineapple is the fruit highest in manganese, an important trace mineral, and along with strawberries, this smoothie delivers a bountiful amount of vitamin C.

> 1 container (4 ounces or 112 g) strawberry low-fat yogurt
> 1/2 cup (120 ml) silken tofu
> 1 package (3 ounces or 85 g) cream cheese, cut into 1/2 -inch (1-cm) pieces
> 1/4 cup (80 g) fruit-only strawberry preserves
> 1/4 cup (32 g) whey protein powder
> 2 tablespoons (30 g) bee pollen
> 1 cup (145 g) strawberries
> 2 cups (310 g) diced pineapple, frozen
> 4 pineapple spears for garnish (optional)

▓ Combine yogurt, tofu, cream cheese, strawberry preserves, whey protein powder, bee pollen, and strawberries in a blender or smoothie maker. Blend on high speed for 45 seconds or until mixture is puréed and smooth. Add pineapple, and blend on high speed again until mixture is smooth. Serve immediately, garnished with pineapple spears, if desired.

▓ **YIELD:** Four 1-cup (235-ml) servings

▓ **NUTRITIONAL ANALYSIS:** Each 1-cup serving provides 260 calories; 9 g total fat; 5 g saturated fat; 13 g protein; 34 g carbohydrate; 3 g dietary fiber; 43 mg cholesterol.

▓ **TIP:** It is a shame to waste a pineapple's leafy crown if you are making a fruit salad or a fruit platter. Once you have sliced it off, slice through the leaves about 2 inches (5 cm) from the base. The pineapple crown then resembles a flower and it becomes an attractive decoration.

SUPERCHARGE NUTRIENTS:	% DAILY VALUE*
Vitamin A	360.9 IU (7%)
Vitamin B6	0.2 mg (8%)
Vitamin C	53.3 mg (89%)
Vitamin E	0.9 mg (5%)
Magnesium	35.7 mg (9%)
Manganese	1.0 mg (51%)
Selenium	2.0 mcg (3%)
Zinc	1.0 mg (7%)

* Percent Daily Values are based on a 2,000 calorie diet. Your daily values may be higher or lower depending on your caloric needs.

WOW FOR WHITE CELLS
PINEAPPLE PEACH APRICOT SMOOTHIE

It is not just tomatoes that have lycopene, a powerful antioxidant; all forms of apricots also deliver this key nutrient. Both apricots and peaches, along with other orange fruits, are also excellent sources of beta-carotene, which your body converts to vitamin A—the vitamin that enhances the function of white blood cells.

> 1 container (8 ounces or 225 g) peach low-fat yogurt
> 1/2 cup (120 ml) silken tofu
> 1/2 cup (65 g) dried apricots
> 1/4 cup (80 g) fruit-only apricot preserves
> 1/4 cup (32 g) whey protein powder
> 2 tablespoons (30 g) bee pollen
> 1 1/2 cups (235 g) diced pineapple
> 1 1/2 cups (255 g) peach slices, frozen
> 4 peach slices for garnish (optional)

■ Combine yogurt, tofu, dried apricots, apricot preserves, whey protein powder, bee pollen, and pineapple in a blender or smoothie maker. Blend on high speed for 45 seconds or until mixture is puréed and smooth. Add peach slices, and blend on high speed again until mixture is smooth. Serve immediately, garnished with peach slices, if desired.

■ **YIELD:** Four 1-cup (235-ml) servings

■ **NUTRITIONAL ANALYSIS:** Each 1-cup serving provides 237 calories; 2 g total fat; 1 g saturated fat; 14 g protein; 45 g carbohydrate; 5 g dietary fiber; 20 mg cholesterol.

■ **TIP:** Fruits like peaches and plums that are irregular in shape are frequently difficult to handle because the stone is not centered. Here is an easy way to handle these fruits: Locate the crease on one side that corresponds to the pointed end of the stone, then slice the fruit at a 90° angle to that crease all the way through the fruit. Then twist the two halves apart and the stone will pop right out.

SUPERCHARGE NUTRIENTS:	% DAILY VALUE*
Vitamin A	2844.1 IU (57%)
Vitamin B6	0.2 mg (9%)
Vitamin C	30.0 mg (50%)
Vitamin E	1.1 mg (6%)
Magnesium	50.2 mg (13%)
Manganese	0.8 mg (42%)
Selenium	2.6 mcg (4%)
Zinc	1.3 mg (9%)

Percent Daily Values are based on a 2,000 calorie diet. Your daily values may be higher or lower depending on your caloric needs.

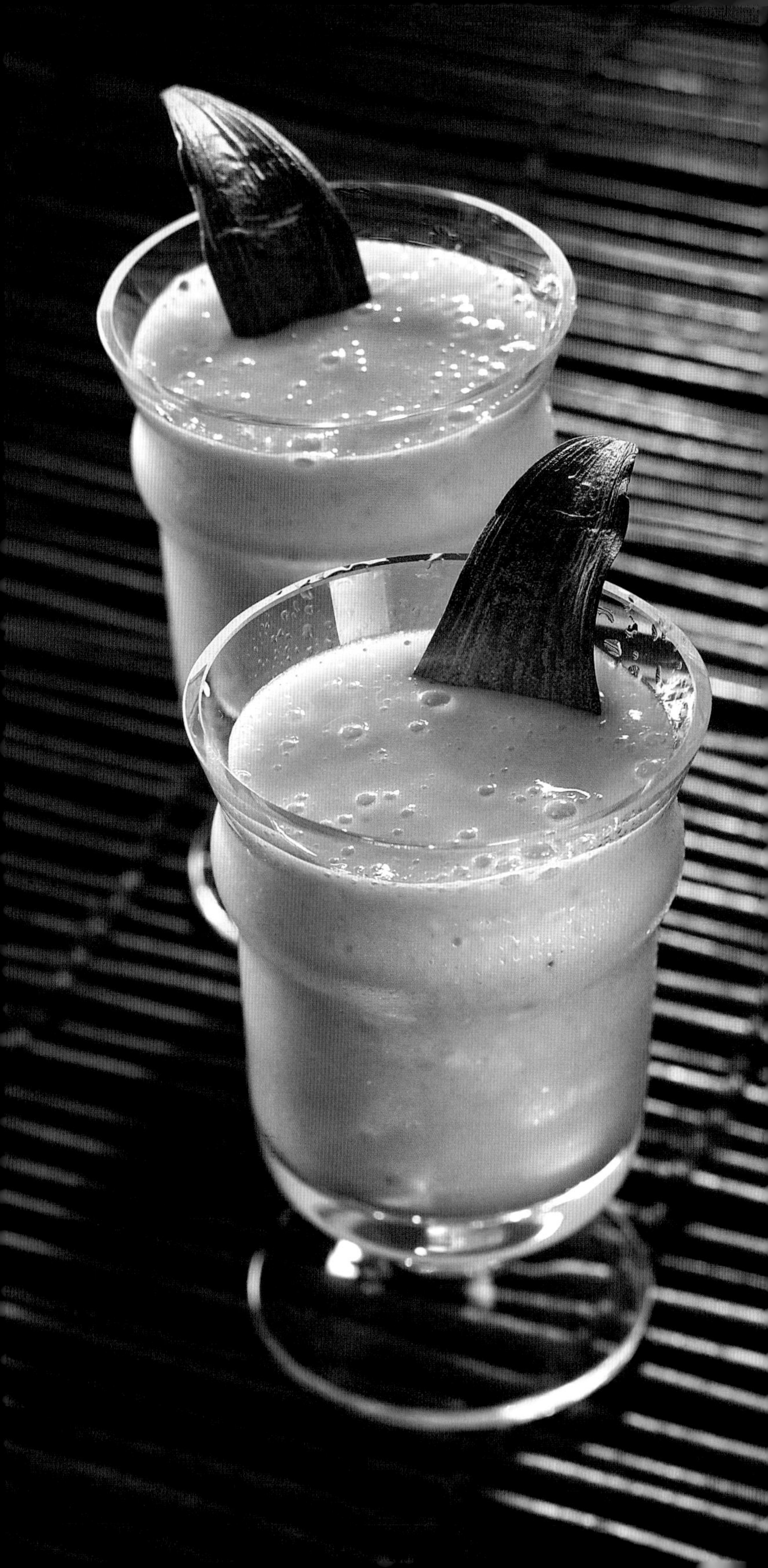

BROMELAIN BONUS
GINGERED PINEAPPLE BANANA SMOOTHIE

In addition to being high in manganese and vitamin C, pineapple is rich in bromelain, an enzyme that aids in digestion and can reduce inflammation. Ginger is also known for its tummy-taming powers, so this luscious tropical smoothie is the one to make if intestinal distress is an issue.

1 cup (235 ml) chilled pineapple juice
$1/2$ cup (120 ml) silken tofu
$1/4$ cup (55 g) crystallized ginger
$1/4$ cup (32 g) whey protein powder
1 cup (155 g) diced pineapple
1 cup (150 g) banana slices, frozen
4 pineapple spears or pineapple leaves for garnish (optional)

▨ Combine pineapple juice, tofu, ginger, whey protein powder, and diced pineapple in a blender or smoothie maker. Blend on high speed for 45 seconds or until mixture is puréed and smooth. Add banana slices, and blend on high speed again until mixture is smooth. Serve immediately, garnished with pineapple spears or leaves, if desired.

▨ **YIELD:** Four 1-cup (235-ml) servings

▨ **NUTRITIONAL ANALYSIS:** Each 1-cup serving provides 193 calories; 1 g total fat; 0 g saturated fat; 8 g protein; 41 g carbohydrate; 2 g dietary fiber; 18 mg cholesterol.

▨ **TIP:** Choosing ripe pineapples and ripe melons can be a challenge because nudging the flesh is not a conclusive test, and flesh that is too soft can mean the fruit is spoiled. I have found that the best test is to smell the fruit at the stem end. If it smells sweet, there is a good chance it is ripe.

SUPERCHARGE NUTRIENTS:	% DAILY VALUE*
Vitamin A	95.0 IU (2%)
Vitamin B6	0.4 mg (21%)
Vitamin C	17.1 mg (29%)
Vitamin E	0.3 mg (1%)
Magnesium	38.1 mg (10%)
Manganese	1.5 mg (74%)
Selenium	2.7 mcg (4%)
Zinc	0.3 mg (2%)

* Percent Daily Values are based on a 2,000 calorie diet. Your daily values may be higher or lower depending on your caloric needs.

BORON BONUS
CRUNCHY RAISIN SMOOTHIE

Boron may not receive a lot of play, but this trace mineral is vital to your health because it prevents bone loss, especially in post-menopausal women. Raisins are an excellent source of boron, and both raisins and their parent fruit—grapes—are very high in antioxidant phenols that boost your immune system.

1 cup (235 ml) plain soy milk
3/4 cup (110 g) raisins
1/2 cup (112 g) shelled sunflower seeds
2 tablespoons (30 ml) flaxseed oil
1/2 teaspoon (2.5 ml) pure vanilla extract
1/4 teaspoon (1.2 g) ground cinnamon
2 cups (320 g) seedless red grapes, frozen
1/4 cup (55 g) granola
2 tablespoons (28 g) granola for garnish (optional)

■ Combine soy milk, raisins, sunflower seeds, flaxseed oil, vanilla extract, and cinnamon in a blender or smoothie maker. Blend on high speed for 45 seconds or until mixture is puréed and smooth. Add grapes, and blend on high speed again until mixture is smooth. Add granola, and pulse a few times to distribute it evenly. Serve immediately, garnished with additional granola, if desired.

■ **YIELD:** Four 1-cup (235-ml) servings

■ **NUTRITIONAL ANALYSIS:** Each 1-cup serving provides 344 calories; 17 g total fat; 2 g saturated fat; 7 g protein; 47 g carbohydrate; 5 g dietary fiber; 0 mg cholesterol.

■ **TIP:** When purchasing small amounts of foods, such as the granola in this recipe or dried coconut in other smoothies, look to the bulk food section of your supermarket or health food store. Make sure to shop at a store that uses closed storage for its bulk foods and that has a brisk business so that bin contents turn over quickly.

SUPERCHARGE NUTRIENTS:	% DAILY VALUE*
Vitamin A	185.1 IU (4%)
Vitamin B6	0.3 mg (14%)
Vitamin C	10.6 mg (18%)
Vitamin E	10.1 mg (51%)
Magnesium	49.2 mg (12%)
Manganese	0.5 mg (24%)
Selenium	13.7 mcg (20%)
Zinc	1.2 mg (8%)

* Percent Daily Values are based on a 2,000 calorie diet. Your daily values may be higher or lower depending on your caloric needs.

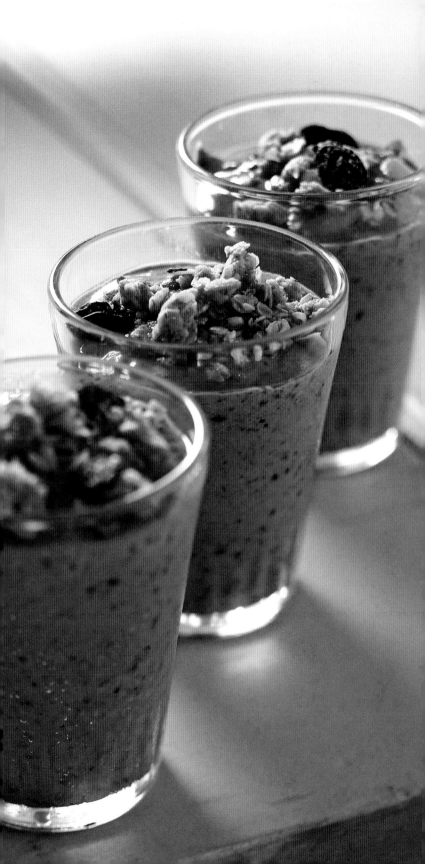

COLON-CONTENT
CARROT RASPBERRY SMOOTHIE

In addition to beta-carotene, carrots also are an excellent source of falcarinol, a phytonutrient that has been shown to reduce the risk of colon cancer. Their sweet flavor is enhanced by that of the raspberries, and both foods are a good source of dietary fiber.

1 container (8 ounces or 225 g) raspberry nonfat yogurt
1/2 cup (120 ml) silken tofu
1/2 cup (120 ml) chilled carrot juice
1/4 cup (80 g) fruit-only raspberry preserves
2 medium carrots, trimmed, scrubbed, and sliced
1/4 cup (32 g) whey protein powder
2 tablespoons (30 ml) flaxseed oil
2 cups (250 g) raspberries, frozen
4 carrot sticks for garnish (optional)

■ Combine yogurt, tofu, carrot juice, raspberry preserves, carrots, whey protein powder, and flaxseed oil in a blender or smoothie maker. Blend on high speed for 45 seconds or until mixture is puréed and smooth. Add raspberries, and blend on high speed again until mixture is smooth. Serve immediately, garnished with carrot sticks, if desired.

■ **YIELD:** Four 1-cup (235-ml) servings

■ **NUTRITIONAL ANALYSIS:** Each 1-cup serving provides 247 calories; 8 g total fat; 1 g saturated fat; 12 g protein; 34 g carbohydrate; 5 g dietary fiber; 20 mg cholesterol.

■ **TIP:** "Baby carrots" in most supermarkets are not really a separate species; they are parts of larger carrots cut by machines into small shapes. Small carrots are inherently sweeter than larger carrots, which tend to be woody. So it is best to buy carrots in bunches and look for small ones.

SUPERCHARGE NUTRIENTS:	% DAILY VALUE*
Vitamin A	12141.9 IU (243%)
Vitamin B6	0.2 mg (8%)
Vitamin C	22.2 mg (37%)
Vitamin E	1.7 mg (9%)
Magnesium	46.9 mg (12%)
Manganese	0.6 mg (28%)
Selenium	2.9 mcg (4%)
Zinc	1.0 mg (7%)

* Percent Daily Values are based on a 2,000 calorie diet. Your daily values may be higher or lower depending on your caloric needs.

BRIGHT EYES
CARROT CITRUS SMOOTHIE

There is no food as high in beta-carotene as bright orange carrots. Once beta-carotene is converted to vitamin A, it helps your eyes by traveling to the retina and transforming into rhodopsin, a purple pigment necessary for night-vision.

> 3 navel oranges
> 1/2 cup (120 ml) chilled carrot juice
> 1/2 cup (120 ml) silken tofu
> 2 medium carrots, trimmed, scrubbed, and sliced
> 1/2 cup (112 g) shelled sunflower seeds
> 1/4 cup (32 g) whey protein powder
> 2 tablespoons (30 ml) flaxseed oil
> 1/2 cup (70 g) orange sherbet
> 1/2 cup (70 g) vanilla frozen yogurt
> 4 carrot sticks for garnish (optional)

▓ Peel oranges, then slice off white pith. Cut around sides of sections to release segments from remaining pith. Cut into 1/2 -inch (1-cm) dice.

▓ Combine oranges, carrot juice, tofu, carrots, sunflower seeds, whey protein powder, and flaxseed oil in a blender or smoothie maker. Blend on high speed for 45 seconds or until mixture is puréed and smooth. Add orange sherbet and frozen yogurt, and blend on high speed again until mixture is smooth. Serve immediately, garnished with carrot sticks, if desired.

▓ **YIELD:** Four 1-cup (235-ml) servings

▓ **NUTRITIONAL ANALYSIS:** Each 1-cup serving provides 315 calories; 17 g total fat; 2 g saturated fat; 13 g protein; 32 g carbohydrate; 5 g dietary fiber; 21 mg cholesterol.

▓ **TIP:** There is really no reason to peel carrots once the skin is scrubbed. If you care to peel them, however, here is an easy way: Pour boiling water over the carrots and allow them to sit for 2 minutes. Plunge them into ice water to cool, and the skins will peel right off.

SUPERCHARGE NUTRIENTS:	% DAILY VALUE*
Vitamin A	12263.2 IU (245%)
Vitamin B6	0.3 mg (15%)
Vitamin C	57.1 mg (95%)
Vitamin E	9.7 mg (48%)
Magnesium	50.8 mg (13%)
Manganese	0.5 mg (23%)
Selenium	14.0 mcg (20%)
Zinc	1.3 mg (9%)

* Percent Daily Values are based on a 2,000 calorie diet. Your daily values may be higher or lower depending on your caloric needs.

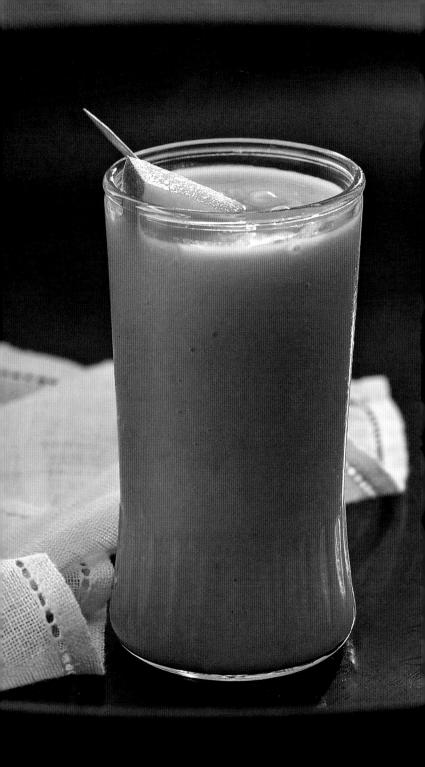

COLON-KIND
PEACHY CARROT SMOOTHIE

In addition to providing tons of beta-carotene to boost your body's supply of vitamin A, carrots contain a phytonutrient called falcarinol, which, according to the *Journal of Agricultural and Food Chemistry*, has been shown to reduce the risk of colon cancer. When carrots are blended into a smoothie with sweet peaches (in three forms), the result is a healthful orange whirl.

> 1 container (8 ounces or 225 g) peach low-fat yogurt
> 1/2 cup (120 ml) chilled carrot juice
> 1/2 cup (120 ml) chilled peach nectar
> 2 medium carrots, trimmed, scrubbed, and sliced
> 2 tablespoons (30 g) bee pollen
> 2 cups (340 g) peach slices, frozen
> 4 fresh peach slices for garnish (optional)

▧ Combine yogurt, carrot juice, peach nectar, carrots, and bee pollen in a blender or smoothie maker. Blend on high speed for 45 seconds or until mixture is puréed and smooth. Add peaches, and blend on high speed again until mixture is smooth. Serve immediately, garnished with fresh peach slices, if desired.

▧ **YIELD:** Four 1-cup (235-ml) servings

▧ **NUTRITIONAL ANALYSIS:** Each 1-cup serving provides 151 calories; 1 g total fat; 1 g saturated fat; 5 g protein; 32 g carbohydrate; 3 g dietary fiber; 2 mg cholesterol.

▧ **TIP:** When buying carrots, try to find bunches with their green leaves still attached. Bright green, perky leaves are a sign that the carrots are fresh. To extend the carrots' life at home, however, cut off the green tops immediately; they rob carrots of nutrients.

SUPERCHARGE NUTRIENTS:	% DAILY VALUE*
Vitamin A	12595.6 IU (252%)
Vitamin B6	0.2 mg (9%)
Vitamin C	25.5 mg (42%)
Vitamin E	1.5 mg (7%)
Magnesium	30.2 mg (8%)
Manganese	0.1 mg (7%)
Selenium	1.2 mcg (2%)
Zinc	1.0 mg (7%)

* Percent Daily Values are based on a 2,000 calorie diet. Your daily values may be higher or lower depending on your caloric needs.

CELL-SUPPORTING GUACAMOLE SMOOTHIE

Avocados are an excellent source of vitamin K, which your body uses for blood clotting. This vitamin also acts as an antioxidant to deactivate free radicals that could damage the delicate fats that are the primary constituents of your cell membranes. In this satisfying and savory smoothie, avocados take center stage, while the other flavors associated with this popular Mexican dip play supporting roles.

> 1 container (8 ounces or 225 g) plain nonfat yogurt
> $1/2$ cup (120 ml) silken tofu
> 2 scallions, trimmed and sliced
> 4 ripe avocados, peeled and diced
> 1 small jalapeño or serrano chile pepper, seeds and ribs removed, and diced
> 2 tablespoons (30 ml) freshly squeezed lime juice
> 2 tablespoons (30 g) bee pollen
> 6 green tea ice cubes
> 4 tortilla chips for garnish (optional)

■ Combine yogurt, tofu, scallions, avocados, chile pepper, lime juice, and bee pollen in a blender or smoothie maker. Blend on high speed for 45 seconds or until mixture is puréed and smooth. Add ice cubes, and blend on high speed again until mixture is smooth. Serve immediately, garnished with tortilla chips, if desired.

■ **YIELD:** Four 1-cup (235-ml) servings

■ **NUTRITIONAL ANALYSIS:** Each 1-cup serving provides 399 calories; 31.5 g total fat; 5 g saturated fat; 9 g protein; 27 g carbohydrate; 11 g dietary fiber; 1 mg cholesterol.

■ **TIP:** It may seem like an oxymoron, but capsicum, the substance that creates the heat in chile peppers, is also an anti-inflammatory and is being studied as an effective treatment for arthritis.

SUPERCHARGE NUTRIENTS:	% DAILY VALUE*
Vitamin A	1318.6 IU (26%)
Vitamin B6	0.6 mg (32%)
Vitamin C	24.3 mg (41%)
Vitamin E	3.3 mg (16%)
Magnesium	96.9 mg (24%)
Manganese	0.5 mg (27%)
Selenium	4.5 mcg (6%)
Zinc	1.8 mg (12%)

Percent Daily Values are based on a 2,000 calorie diet. Your daily values may be higher or lower depending on your caloric needs.

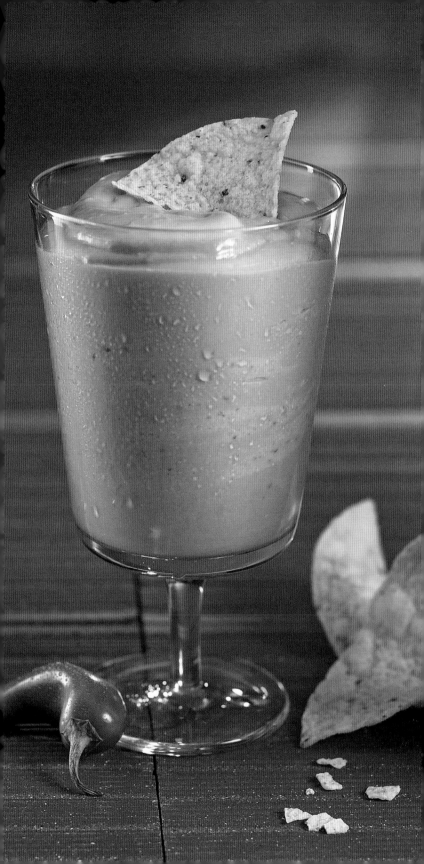

MINERAL MAGIC
AVOCADO RASPBERRY SESAME SMOOTHIE

Avocados add a creamy richness to smoothies, and this buttery texture is a perfect foil for the tart flavor of raspberries and the heady aroma of sesame from the tahini. Sesame also adds a number of vital minerals to the frosty glass, including copper, which is incorporated into a compound called ceruloplasmin, an enzyme that facilitates the oxidation of minerals.

1 container (8 ounces or 225 g) plain nonfat yogurt
$1/2$ cup (120 ml) silken tofu
4 ripe avocados, peeled and diced
$1/3$ cup (80 g) tahini
$1/4$ cup (32 g) whey protein powder
2 tablespoons (30 g) bee pollen
1 $1/2$ cups (190 g) raspberries, frozen
2 tablespoons (15 g) toasted sesame seeds for garnish (optional)

▓ Combine yogurt, tofu, avocados, tahini, whey protein powder, and bee pollen in a blender or smoothie maker. Blend on high speed for 45 seconds or until mixture is puréed and smooth. Add raspberries, and blend on high speed again until mixture is smooth. Serve immediately, garnished with sesame seeds, if desired.

▓ **YIELD:** Four 1-cup (235-ml) servings

▓ **NUTRITIONAL ANALYSIS:** Each 1-cup serving provides 555 calories; 35 g total fat; 5 g saturated fat; 19 g protein; 51.5 g carbohydrate; 19 g dietary fiber; 19.5 mg cholesterol.

▓ **TIP:** A soft avocado can be bruised rather than ripe. One test is to flick off the small stem from the narrow end of the fruit. If it comes off easily and you can see green flesh below, then the avocado is ripe. If it is hard to remove the avocado is not ripe, and if the flesh below is brown, the avocado is bruised.

SUPERCHARGE NUTRIENTS:	% DAILY VALUE*
Vitamin A	1310.7 IU (26%)
Vitamin B6	0.6 mg (31%)
Vitamin C	39.9 mg (66%)
Vitamin E	3.4 mg (17%)
Magnesium	98.6 mg (25%)
Manganese	1.0 mg (50%)
Selenium	3.2 mcg (5%)
Zinc	2.7 mg (18%)

* Percent Daily Values are based on a 2,000 calorie diet. Your daily values may be higher or lower depending on your caloric needs.

A-BETA-C
AVOCADO MANGO PAPAYA SMOOTHIE

Tropical fruits like mango and papaya were meant to be enjoyed together, and both are treasure-troves of vitamins C, as well as beta-carotene, which your body converts into vitamin A. The buttery richness of avocado also adds its mineral bounty of potassium and folate to this smoothie.

> 1 container (8 ounces or 225 g) lemon nonfat yogurt
> 1/2 cup (120 ml) silken tofu
> 1 cup (175 g) diced mango
> 2 ripe avocados, peeled and diced
> 1/4 cup (56 g) shelled sunflower seeds
> 1/4 cup (32 g) whey protein powder
> 1/4 cup (32 g) crystallized ginger
> 2 cups (280 g) papaya cubes, frozen
> 4 papaya spears for garnish (optional)

▓ Combine yogurt, tofu, mango, avocados, sunflower seeds, whey protein powder, and ginger in a blender or smoothie maker. Blend on high speed for 45 seconds or until mixture is puréed and smooth. Add papaya cubes, and blend on high speed again until mixture is smooth. Serve immediately, garnished with papaya spears, if desired.

▓ **YIELD:** Four 1-cup (235-ml) servings

▓ **NUTRITIONAL ANALYSIS:** Each 1-cup serving provides 359 calories; 20 g total fat; 3 g saturated fat; 15 g protein; 36 g carbohydrate; 10 g dietary fiber; 19.5 mg cholesterol.

▓ **TIP:** Mangoes are notoriously hard to peel because of their irregular shape. Peeling them is easier if you cut a small slice off the larger end, and then stand the mango up on the cut surface. Then peel from top to bottom.

SUPERCHARGE NUTRIENTS:	% DAILY VALUE*
Vitamin A	3651.0 IU (73%)
Vitamin B6	0.4 mg (21%)
Vitamin C	65.4 mg (109%)
Vitamin E	6.6 mg (33%)
Magnesium	68.0 mg (17%)
Manganese	0.3 mg (17%)
Selenium	9.5 mcg (14%)
Zinc	1.7 mg (11%)

* Percent Daily Values are based on a 2,000 calorie diet. Your daily values may be higher or lower depending on your caloric needs.

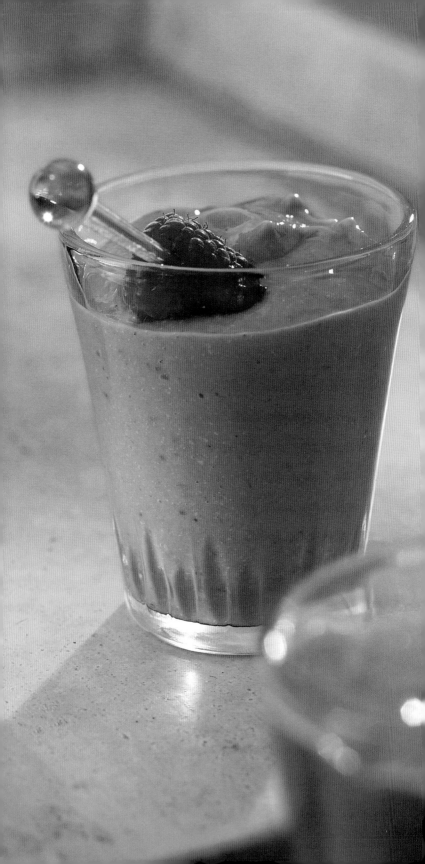

BLOOD-BOOSTING
GRAPEFRUIT AVOCADO SMOOTHIE

The body uses vitamin K, found in abundance in avocados, to help the blood coagulate properly and form clots when we are injured; these clots then protect the skin from being penetrated by micro-organisms. A good source of fiber, potassium, and folate, avocados add richness to this purée of vitamin C-rich grapefruit and sweet raspberries.

> 2 red grapefruit
> 1/2 cup (120 ml) freshly squeezed orange juice
> 1/2 cup (120 ml) silken tofu
> 1/4 cup (56 g) shelled sunflower seeds
> 2 ripe avocados, peeled and diced
> 1/2 cup (65 g) raspberries, frozen
> 4 green tea ice cubes
> 4 raspberries or grapefruit sections reserved for garnish (optional)

▓ Peel grapefruit and slice off white pith. Cut around sides of sections to release segments from remaining pith. Reserve four sections, if using as garnish, and cut remaining grapefruit into 1/2-inch (1-cm) dice.

▓ Combine grapefruit sections, orange juice, tofu, sunflower seeds, and avocados in a blender or smoothie maker. Blend on high speed for 45 seconds or until mixture is puréed and smooth. Add frozen raspberries and ice cubes, and blend on high speed again until mixture is smooth. Serve immediately, garnished with grapefruit sections, if desired.

▓ **YIELD:** Four 1-cup (235-ml) servings

▓ **NUTRITIONAL ANALYSIS:** Each 1-cup serving provides 277 calories; 20 g total fat; 3 g saturated fat; 5 g protein; 25 g carbohydrate; 7 g dietary fiber; 0 mg cholesterol.

▓ **TIP:** Avocados are rich in nutrients and an excellent source of oleic acid, a monounsaturated fat that may help lower cholesterol. Try puréeing avocados (in place of olive oil) with vinegar and spices as a tasty way to add nutrients to salad dressing.

SUPERCHARGE NUTRIENTS:	% DAILY VALUE*
Vitamin A	1015.6 IU (20%)
Vitamin B6	0.4 mg (22%)
Vitamin C	72.9 mg (121%)
Vitamin E	5.8 mg (29%)
Magnesium	69.3 mg (17%)
Manganese	0.6 mg (31%)
Selenium	10.1 mcg (14%)
Zinc	1.1 mg (7%)

* Percent Daily Values are based on a 2,000 calorie diet. Your daily values may be higher or lower depending on your caloric needs.

FLOW WITH THE FLAVONOIDS
APPLE AVOCADO SMOOTHIE

Both apples and avocados have a mildly sweet flavor, and a good amount of antioxidant flavonoids. The sunflower seeds add crunchy texture, along with a high content of vitamin E and minerals.

1 cup (235 ml) cloudy apple juice, chilled
$1/2$ cup (120 ml) silken tofu
2 sweet eating apples (such as McIntosh or Red Delicious),
    cored and diced
1 ripe avocado, peeled and diced
$1/2$ cup (112 g) shelled sunflower seeds
$1/4$ cup (32 g) whey protein powder
2 tablespoons (40 g) honey
8 green tea ice cubes
4 apple wedges for garnish (optional)

▨ Combine apple juice, tofu, apples, avocado, sunflower seeds, whey protein powder, and honey in a blender or smoothie maker. Blend on high speed for 45 seconds or until mixture is puréed and smooth. Add ice cubes, and blend on high speed again until mixture is smooth. Serve immediately, garnished with apple wedges, if desired.

▨ **YIELD:** Four 1-cup (235-ml) servings

▨ **NUTRITIONAL ANALYSIS:** Each 1-cup serving provides 313 calories; 16 g total fat; 2 g saturated fat; 12 g protein; 35 g carbohydrate; 6 g dietary fiber; 18 mg cholesterol.

▨ **TIP:** If you are slicing apples for a tart, then making the slices decorative is a goal. However, if you are prepping them for a smoothie, there is no reason to go to any trouble for the sake of appearance. Just slice off hunks from the outside, and when you get to the core, discard it.

SUPERCHARGE NUTRIENTS:	% DAILY VALUE*
Vitamin A	360.7 IU (7%)
Vitamin B6	0.3 mg (15%)
Vitamin C	9.1 mg (15%)
Vitamin E	9.1 mg (46%)
Magnesium	46.2 mg (12%)
Manganese	0.5 mg (26%)
Selenium	13.0 mcg (19%)
Zinc	1.3 mg (9%)

Percent Daily Values are based on a 2,000 calorie diet. Your daily values may be higher or lower depending on your caloric needs.

CRUNCHY K-ZONE
APPLE ALMOND CELERY SMOOTHIE

Vitamin K is very necessary for your body to promote blood clotting, and while avocado is an excellent source, there is also some in celery—and for far fewer calories! The mild taste of celery allows the sweetness of flavonoid-filled apples and protein-rich almonds to blend harmoniously in this smoothie.

> 1 cup (235 ml) cloudy apple juice
> 1 container (8 ounces or 225 g) lemon nonfat yogurt
> 2 cups (200 g) diced celery
> 2 Granny Smith apples, cored, and diced
> 1/2 cup (75 g) shelled almonds, not skinned
> 1/4 cup (32 g) whey protein powder
> 1/4 cup (65 g) apple chutney
> 3 tablespoons (45 ml) flaxseed oil
> 4 celery sticks for garnish (optional)

▦ Pour apple juice into ice cube tray, and freeze until solid.

▦ Combine yogurt, celery, apples, almonds, whey protein powder, apple chutney, and flaxseed oil in a blender or smoothie maker. Blend on high speed for 45 seconds or until mixture is puréed and smooth. Add apple juice cubes, and blend on high speed again until mixture is smooth. Serve immediately, garnished with celery sticks, if desired.

▦ **YIELD:** Four 1-cup (235-ml) servings

▦ **NUTRITIONAL ANALYSIS:** Each 1-cup serving provides 342 calories; 20 g total fat; 2 g saturated fat; 14 g protein; 32 g carbohydrate; 4.5 g dietary fiber; 19.5 mg cholesterol.

▦ **TIP:** Any fruit juice can be turned into ice cubes, and these cubes are very versatile for more than smoothies. Use apple juice cubes in iced tea to sweeten as well as cool it, or orange juice cubes in sparkling water.

SUPERCHARGE NUTRIENTS:	% DAILY VALUE*
Vitamin A	242.5 IU (5%)
Vitamin B6	0.2 mg (8%)
Vitamin C	14.0 mg (23%)
Vitamin E	6.7 mg (34%)
Magnesium	78.1 mg (20%)
Manganese	0.6 mg (30%)
Selenium	2.5 mcg (4%)
Zinc	1.2 mg (8%)

* Percent Daily Values are based on a 2,000 calorie diet. Your daily values may be higher or lower depending on your caloric needs.

BETA-BLAST
CANTALOUPE GAZPACHO SMOOTHIE

Cantaloupe's orange color should be your clue that this low-calorie fruit is loaded with beta-carotene, which our bodies turn into vitamin A, an important antioxidant. This smoothie also contains lycopene-laden orange tomatoes and other vegetables, and its flavor—while basically sweet—has hot and sour notes as well.

1 container (8 ounces or 225 g) plain nonfat yogurt
1/2 cup (120 ml) silken tofu
1/2 pound (225 g) orange tomatoes, cored, and cut into 1-inch (2.5-cm) cubes
1/2 small orange bell pepper, seeds and ribs removed, and diced
1 celery stalk, trimmed and sliced
1 small shallot, peeled and sliced
2 tablespoons (30 ml) cider vinegar
2 tablespoons (30 ml) flaxseed oil
2 cups (310 g) diced cantaloupe, frozen
Salt and hot pepper sauce to taste
4 celery sprigs for garnish (optional)

■ Combine yogurt, tofu, tomatoes, bell pepper, celery, shallot, vinegar, and flaxseed oil in a blender or smoothie maker. Blend on high speed for 45 seconds or until mixture is puréed and smooth. Add cantaloupe, and blend on high speed again until mixture is smooth. Season to taste with salt and hot pepper sauce, and serve immediately, garnished with celery sprigs, if desired.

■ **YIELD:** Four 1-cup (235-ml) servings

■ **NUTRITIONAL ANALYSIS:** Each 1-cup serving provides 142 calories; 8 g total fat; 1 g saturated fat; 5.5 g protein; 15 g carbohydrate; 1.5 g dietary fiber; 1 mg cholesterol.

■ **TIP:** If you would rather serve this as a refreshing summer soup, use chilled cantaloupe instead of frozen.

SUPERCHARGE NUTRIENTS:	% DAILY VALUE*
Vitamin A	3925.9 IU (79%)
Vitamin B6	0.2 mg (10%)
Vitamin C	72.6 mg (121%)
Vitamin E	2.8 mg (14%)
Magnesium	35.4 mg (9%)
Manganese	0.1 mg (6%)
Selenium	2.7 mcg (4%)
Zinc	0.7 mg (4%)

* Percent Daily Values are based on a 2,000 calorie diet. Your daily values may be higher or lower depending on your caloric needs.

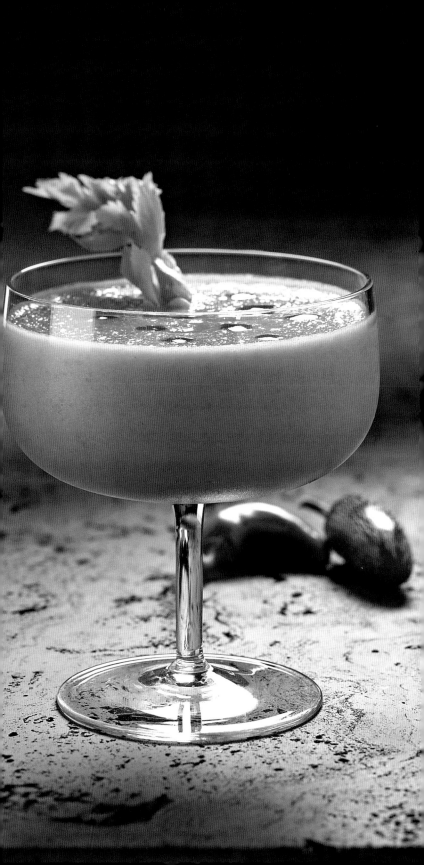

MARVEL AT THE MANGANESE PINEAPPLE GAZPACHO SMOOTHIE

No fruit offers you as much manganese, a trace mineral that is part of many of your body's needed enzymes, as pineapple. Its sweet and tart flavor blends well with vegetables such as mild bell peppers.

> 1 cup (235 ml) pineapple juice, chilled
> 1 container (8 ounces or 225 g) pineapple nonfat yogurt
> 1/2 medium cucumber, peeled, seeded, and diced
> 1/2 medium yellow bell pepper, seeds and ribs removed, and diced
> 1 small jalapeño or serrano chile, seeds and ribs removed, and diced
> 2 scallions, white part only, rinsed, trimmed, and sliced
> 1/4 cup (32 g) whey protein powder
> 3 tablespoons (45 ml) flaxseed oil
> 2 tablespoons (30 ml) freshly squeezed lime juice
> 1 1/2 cups (250 g) pineapple cubes, frozen
> 4 pineapple spears for garnish (optional)

■ Combine pineapple juice, yogurt, cucumber, bell pepper, chile pepper, scallions, whey protein powder, flaxseed oil, and lime juice a blender or smoothie maker. Blend on high speed for 45 seconds or until mixture is puréed and smooth. Add pineapple cubes, and blend on high speed again until mixture is smooth. Serve immediately, garnished with pineapple spears, if desired.

■ **YIELD:** Four 1-cup (235-ml) servings

■ **NUTRITIONAL ANALYSIS:** Each 1-cup serving provides 227 calories; 10.5 g total fat; 1 g saturated fat; 11 g protein; 24.5 g carbohydrate; 2 g dietary fiber; 19.5 mg cholesterol.

■ **TIP:** Most recipes call for the seeds and ribs to be removed from bell peppers. Here is a quick and easy way: Cut a slice off the bottom of the pepper so that it sits firmly on the counter. Then cut down the bulges of the pepper. Simply discard the core of seeds and ribs.

SUPERCHARGE NUTRIENTS:	% DAILY VALUE*
Vitamin A	198.0 IU (4%)
Vitamin B6	0.2 mg (12%)
Vitamin C	76.8 mg (128%)
Vitamin E	1.8 mg (9%)
Magnesium	39.1 mg (10%)
Manganese	1.1 mg (54%)
Selenium	2.4 mcg (3%)
Zinc	0.8 mg (6%)

* Percent Daily Values are based on a 2,000 calorie diet. Your daily values may be higher or lower depending on your caloric needs.

ADVANTAGE TO THE A-TEAM MANGO GAZPACHO SMOOTHIE

Cucumbers are related to watermelons and zucchini. One health benefit they add to smoothies is that they are a source of vitamin C, as well as the minerals manganese and folate.

1 container (8 ounces or 225 g) plain nonfat yogurt
$1/2$ cup (120 ml) silken tofu
$1/2$ cup (120 ml) freshly squeezed orange juice, chilled
1 celery stalk, rinsed and diced
$1/2$ small cucumber, peeled, seeded, and diced
1 sweet red eating apple (such as McIntosh or Red Delicious),
    cored and diced
$1/4$ cup (32 g) whey protein powder
2 tablespoons (30 ml) flaxseed oil
1 tablespoon (8 g) crystallized ginger
1 tablespoon (15 ml) freshly squeezed lime juice
2 cups (280 g) mango cubes, frozen
4 mango spears for garnish (optional)

▨ Combine yogurt, tofu, orange juice, celery, cucumber, apple, whey protein powder, flaxseed oil, ginger, and lime juice in a blender or smoothie maker. Blend on high speed for 45 seconds or until mixture is puréed and smooth. Add mango cubes, and blend on high speed again until mixture is smooth. Serve immediately, garnished with mango spears, if desired.

▨ **YIELD:** Four 1-cup (235-ml) servings

▨ **NUTRITIONAL ANALYSIS:** Each 1-cup serving provides 224 calories; 8 g total fat; 1 g saturated fat; 11 g protein; 30.5 g carbohydrate; 3 g dietary fiber; 19.5 mg cholesterol.

▨ **TIP:** If you purchase organic cucumbers, there's no need to peel them; just scrub them well to remove any dirt on the surface. Most commercial cucumbers, however, have been coated with wax to prevent bruising and drying out during shipping and must be peeled.

SUPERCHARGE NUTRIENTS:	% DAILY VALUE*
Vitamin A	3397.5 IU (68%)
Vitamin B6	0.2 mg (10%)
Vitamin C	43.0 mg (72%)
Vitamin E	2.3 mg (12%)
Magnesium	33.8 mg (8%)
Manganese	0.1 mg (4%)
Selenium	2.7 mcg (4%)
Zinc	0.6 mg (4%)

* Percent Daily Values are based on a 2,000 calorie diet. Your daily values may be higher or lower depending on your caloric needs.

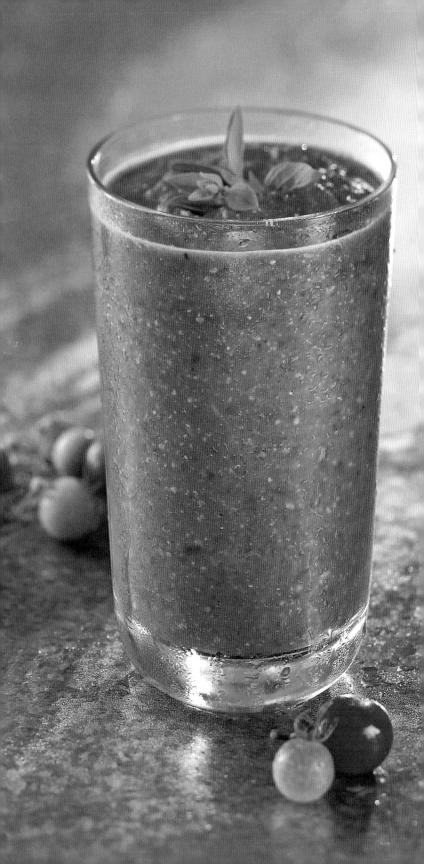

TERRIFIC THIAMIN
HERBED TOMATO SMOOTHIE

Maintaining your body's energy supply is fundamental in keeping your immune system healthy, and that is where vitamin B1, commonly called thiamin, comes in. Sunflower seeds are a superb source of this key nutrient. The seeds add a crunchy texture to this savory smoothie that also delivers heart-protecting lycopene from the tomatoes.

> 1 cup (235 ml) chilled tomato juice
> 2/3 cup (150 g) shelled sunflower seeds
> 1/4 cup (32 g) whey protein powder
> 1 tablespoon (15 ml) freshly squeezed lemon juice
> 1/2 cup (20 g) loosely packed fresh basil leaves
> 1/4 cup (10 g) loosely packed fresh oregano leaves
> 1/4 cup (15 g) loosely packed fresh parsley leaves
> 1 pound (455 g) fresh tomatoes, cored, diced, and frozen
> Salt and freshly ground black pepper to taste
> 4 herb sprigs for garnish (optional)

■ Combine tomato juice, sunflower seeds, whey protein powder, lemon juice, basil, oregano, and parsley in a blender or smoothie maker. Blend on high speed for 45 seconds or until mixture is puréed and smooth. Add tomatoes, and blend on high speed again until mixture is smooth. Season to taste with salt and pepper. Serve immediately, garnished with herb sprigs, if desired.

■ **YIELD:** Four 1-cup (235-ml) servings

■ **NUTRITIONAL ANALYSIS:** Each 1-cup serving provides 205 calories; 12 g total fat; 2 g saturated fat; 13 g protein; 17 g carbohydrate; 6 g dietary fiber; 18 mg cholesterol.

■ **TIP:** There's nothing better than tomato juice that you make yourself, and it is easy with a blender or food processor. Simply purée the tomatoes and then strain out the pulp. (If you were to use the pulp, the smoothie would be too thick to drink.)

SUPERCHARGE NUTRIENTS:	% DAILY VALUE*
Vitamin A	1527.8 IU (31%)
Vitamin B6	0.4 mg (20%)
Vitamin C	34.2 mg (57%)
Vitamin E	11.9 mg (59%)
Magnesium	67.7 mg (17%)
Manganese	0.9 mg (45%)
Selenium	17.8 mcg (25%)
Zinc	1.6 mg (10%)

Percent Daily Values are based on a 2,000 calorie diet. Your daily values may be higher or lower depending on your caloric needs.

CONTENT CAROTENES
PEACH GAZPACHO SMOOTHIE

While gazpacho is a classic cold soup from Spain, it has become a genre—like salsa—for any thick cold soup that has vegetables and, in many cases, fruit. The peach slices deliver a wonderful dose of beta-carotene, which your body converts into vitamin A, and the flaxseed oil is a good source of omega-3 fatty acids, which can help to boost your immune system.

> 1 container (8 ounces or 225 g) plain nonfat yogurt
> 1/2 cup (120 ml) silken tofu
> 2 cups (360 g) diced orange tomatoes
> 1 shallot, peeled and diced
> 1/4 cup (32 g) whey protein powder
> 3 tablespoons (45 ml) flaxseed oil
> 2 tablespoons (30 ml) cider vinegar
> 2 cups (340 g) peach slices, frozen
> Salt and freshly ground pepper to taste
> 4 peach slices for garnish (optional)

Combine yogurt, tofu, tomatoes, shallot, whey protein powder, flaxseed oil, and cider vinegar in a blender or smoothie maker. Blend on high speed for 45 seconds or until mixture is puréed and smooth. Add peach slices, and blend on high speed again until mixture is smooth. Season to taste with salt and pepper. Serve immediately, garnished with peach slices, if desired.

YIELD: Four 1-cup (235-ml) servings

NUTRITIONAL ANALYSIS: Each 1-cup serving provides 207 calories; 11 g total fat; 1 g saturated fat; 13 g protein; 16.5 g carbohydrate; 2 g dietary fiber; 19.5 mg cholesterol.

TIP: If you want to use flaxseeds rather than the oil pressed from them, they will add a bit more nuttiness to the flavor of your smoothie. Use 2 tablespoons (30 g) of seeds for each 1 tablespoon (15 ml) of oil, and grind the seeds in the blender before adding any other ingredients.

SUPERCHARGE NUTRIENTS:	% DAILY VALUE*
Vitamin A	1663.1 IU (33%)
Vitamin B6	0.1 mg (5%)
Vitamin C	18.9 mg (32%)
Vitamin E	2.3 mg (12%)
Magnesium	33.7 mg (8%)
Manganese	0.1 mg (6%)
Selenium	2.5 mcg (4%)
Zinc	0.8 mg (5%)

* Percent Daily Values are based on a 2,000 calorie diet. Your daily values may be higher or lower depending on your caloric needs.

NORTH AFRICAN-SPICED
E-XCELLENT TOMATO SMOOTHIE

Traditional North African spices enliven the flavor of this lycopene-rich tomato smoothie. The sunflower seeds add vitamin E and vitamin B1 to the immune-boosting mix.

- 3/4 cup (175 ml) tomato juice, chilled
- 1 pound (455 g) ripe tomatoes, cored and diced
- 1 shallot, peeled and diced
- 1 large garlic clove, peeled
- 1/2 cup (112 g) shelled sunflower seeds
- 2 sprigs fresh parsley
- 2 sprigs fresh cilantro
- 1/4 cup (32 g) whey protein powder
- 1 tablespoon (20 g) honey
- 2 teaspoons (10 ml) freshly squeezed lemon juice
- 1 teaspoon (5 g) paprika
- 1 teaspoon (5 g) ground cumin
- 1/2 teaspoon (1 g) ground ginger
- 1/2 teaspoon (1.2 g) ground cinnamon
- 6 green tea ice cubes
- Salt and freshly ground pepper to taste
- 4 lemon slices for garnish (optional)

■ Combine all but the last 3 ingredients in a blender or smoothie maker. Blend on high speed for 45 seconds or until mixture is puréed and smooth. Add ice cubes, and blend on high speed again until mixture is smooth. Season to taste with salt and pepper. Serve immediately, garnished with lemon slices, if desired.

■ **YIELD:** Four 1-cup (235-ml) servings

■ **NUTRITIONAL ANALYSIS:** Each 1-cup serving provides 174 calories; 9 g total fat; 1 g saturated fat; 11 g protein; 16 g carbohydrate; 4 g dietary fiber; 18 mg cholesterol.

■ **TIP:** I like using shallots in smoothies because their flavor is more gentle than that of onions. Scallions are the best alternative to shallots.

SUPERCHARGE NUTRIENTS:	% DAILY VALUE*
Vitamin A	1318.7 IU (26%)
Vitamin B6	0.3 mg (15%)
Vitamin C	20.9 mg (35%)
Vitamin E	8.9 mg (44%)
Magnesium	44.0 mg (11%)
Manganese	0.6 mg (32%)
Selenium	13.1 mcg (19%)
Zinc	1.2 mg (8%)

* Percent Daily Values are based on a 2,000 calorie diet. Your daily values may be higher or lower depending on your caloric needs.

LYCOPENE LUSTER
TOMATO CARROT SMOOTHIE

Lycopene, a phytonutrient found in tomatoes, is a powerful antioxidant; you can recognize it in tomatoes' deep red color. When joined with equally sweet carrots and seasoned with savory flavors including healthful garlic, this smoothie is a refreshing treat.

   $^1/_2$ cup (120 ml) chilled carrot juice
   $^1/_2$ cup (120 ml) chilled tomato juice
   1 small carrot, scrubbed and sliced
   2 scallions, trimmed and sliced
   3 tablespoons (12 g) fresh cilantro leaves
   2 tablespoons (28 ml) rice vinegar
   2 tablespoons (30 ml) flaxseed oil
   1 tablespoon (15 ml) reduced-sodium soy sauce
   1 garlic clove, peeled
   1 $^1/_4$ cups (225 g) diced tomatoes, frozen
   Freshly ground black pepper to taste
   4 carrot sticks or cilantro sprigs for garnish (optional)

■ Combine carrot juice, tomato juice, carrot, scallions, cilantro leaves, rice vinegar, flaxseed oil, soy sauce, and garlic in a blender or smoothie maker. Blend on high speed for 45 seconds or until mixture is puréed and smooth. Add tomatoes, and blend on high speed again until mixture is smooth. Season to taste with pepper, and serve immediately, garnished with carrot sticks, if desired.

■ **YIELD:** Four 1-cup (235-ml) servings

■ **NUTRITIONAL ANALYSIS:** Each 1-cup serving provides 100 calories; 7 g total fat; 1 g saturated fat; 2 g protein; 9 g carbohydrate; 2 g dietary fiber; 0 mg cholesterol.

■ **TIP:** Cilantro, like parsley and dill, is a tender herb that wilts quickly once it is picked. A way to extend its life is to trim the stems and refrigerate the herb standing upright in a glass of water. The stems will absorb water like cut flowers and stay perky for up to a week.

SUPERCHARGE NUTRIENTS:	% DAILY VALUE*
Vitamin A	7151.6 IU (143%)
Vitamin B6	0.2 mg (9%)
Vitamin C	19.0 mg (32%)
Vitamin E	1.9 mg (9%)
Magnesium	21.7 mg (5%)
Manganese	0.2 mg (10%)
Selenium	1.1 mcg (2%)
Zinc	0.2 mg (2%)

Percent Daily Values are based on a 2,000 calorie diet. Your daily values may be higher or lower depending on your caloric needs.

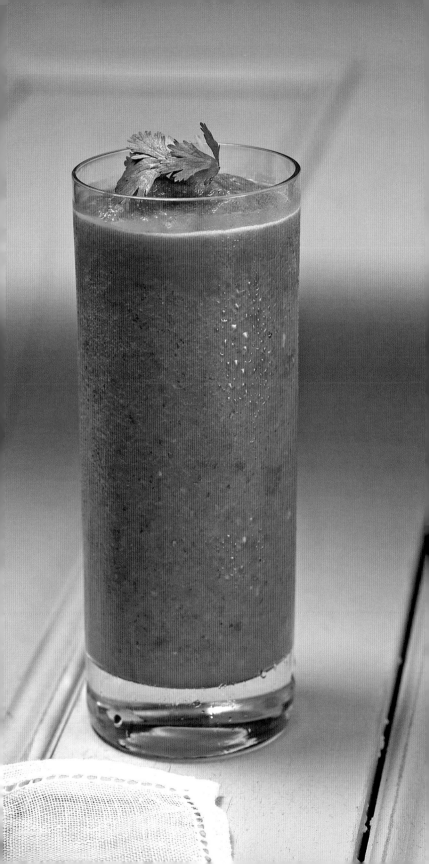

GLOSSARY

A

acidophilus: A friendly bacteria, used to thicken yogurt, that helps prevent intestinal infections.

amino acids: The building blocks of proteins. Humans can produce ten of the twenty amino acids we need; the remainder must come from the foods we eat.

antigen: A foreign substance capable of stimulating an immune response.

antioxidant: A substance that can inhibit the damaging effects of free radicals.

autoimmune disease: A disease caused by the body's immune system attacking its own tissues.

B

bee pollen: A protein-rich honey by-product made from the seeds of flower blossoms.

binder: A thickening ingredient such as banana or egg yolks.

boron: A trace mineral that inhibits bone loss.

bromelain: An enzyme found only in pineapple that breaks down proteins and has anti-inflammatory properties.

C

calcium: A mineral found mainly in the hard part of bones.

carotenoid: A compound in fruits and vegetables that the body converts to vitamin A.

catechin: An antioxidant found in chocolate and green tea.

copper: A trace mineral that plays a role in the formation of many enzymes.

D

dry-packed: How fruit is described when it is frozen in individual pieces without added sugar or syrup.

E

ellagic acid: A phytonutrient found in raspberries, blueberries, strawberries, and blackberries.

emulsion: A combination of two ingredients of different compositions blended to form a new mixture.

enzyme: A protein that acts as a catalyst to induce chemical changes in the body.

extract: A liquid whose flavor is highly concentrated by distillation or evaporation.

F

flavonoid: A subset of polyphenols that act as antioxidants and consist of thousands of compounds responsible for the color of plants.

flaxseed: The small seed of flax, also called linseed, that has a nutty flavor and contains omega-3 fatty acids.

folate: One of the B vitamins that is key to making nucleic acid for DNA. (Also called folic acid.)

free radical: A highly reactive chemical form that can damage cells in the body and lead to illness (although it is a natural part of the metabolic process).

G

garnish: An embellishment added to a dish to enhance its visual appeal.

glutamine: An amino acid that helps keep the body's acid-base ratio in balance.

grate: To shave into tiny pieces using a sharp rasp or grater.

I

immune system: The system of internal defense mechanisms that enables the body to resist and fight disease.

infusion: A liquid in which ingredients such as herbs have been soaked or steeped to extract flavor into the liquid.

iron: The mineral that serves as the core of red blood cells.

L

lipoic acid: An antioxidant that deactivates free radicals and strengthens the effects of other antioxidants such as vitamins C and E.

lycopene: The red pigment found in tomatoes and raspberries that gives them their color and has powerful antioxidant properties.

lymphoid organs: The series of organs, including the spleen, lymph nodes, and bone marrow, that operate with the lymphoid vessels to create the immune system.

M

magnesium: A mineral that is the cofactor (or helping molecule) for approximately 350 enzymes involved in many processes.

manganese: The main antioxidant enzyme in the mitochondria, the cell's power producers.

N

nectar: A juice made from tree fruits such as peaches and apricots that has a thicker consistency than regular fruit juice.

O

omega-3: A fatty acid in cells' membranes that activates an enzyme that suppresses tumor growth and acts to lower cholesterol levels.

P

papain: An enzyme found in the skin of papaya that helps relieve indigestion (and tenderizes meats when used as part of a marinade).

pathogen: Any bacteria, virus, parasite, or fungus that infects the body and triggers an immune response.

phytonutrient: Plant compounds that have health-promoting qualities.

polyphenols: A group of phytonutrients found in certain fruits and nuts, tea, red wine, and cocoa that act as an antioxidant.

potassium: A mineral necessary for proper cell function.

protein: A large molecule made from one or more chains of amino acids.

purée: To reduce food to a thick, creamy texture, typically by using a blender or food processor.

R

resveratrol: An antioxidant found in grapes, peanuts, and red wine that is thought to prevent heart disease.

S

selenium: A trace mineral that acts as an antioxidant.

sorbet: A fruit-flavored ice made without dairy products.

T

tahini: A paste made from sesame seeds that is used to flavor many Middle Eastern dishes.

tofu: A protein-rich substance made from soybeans and soy milk.

twist: A thin strip of citrus zest folded into a decorative shape.

U

unsulphured dry fruit: Dried fruit that has not been sprayed with sulphur dioxide, a gas used for fumigation that destroys B vitamins.

W

whey protein powder: A substance derived from the by-product of cheese-making that contains protein and amino acids.

Y

yogurt: A coagulated milk product made with friendly bacteria that causes the milk to thicken and gives it a tangy, slightly astringent taste.

Z

zest: Small slivers of citrus peel.

zinc: A mineral involved in protein synthesis and cell division.

ACKNOWLEDGMENTS

Writing a book is a solitary endeavor but its publication is a team effort. I would like to thank Jill Alexander of Fair Winds Press for envisioning the idea for this book, and Ed Claflin, my agent, for his constant encouragement. I also want to thank Nancy King and Amanda Waddell for their editorial assistance, and most importantly, I want to thank Karen Konopelski, nutritionist *extraordinaire*, for all of her guidance and knowledge on human nutrition in general and the immune system in particular. And—as with every book I write—I must thank my feline muses, Tigger-Cat Brown and Patches-Kitten Brown, for keeping me company at the computer and in the kitchen.

—Ellen Brown

ABOUT THE AUTHORS

Ellen Brown is the founding food editor of *USA Today* and the author of eighteen cookbooks, including the award-winning *Gourmet Gazelle Cookbook*, which appeared on the *Cook's Illustrated* best-seller list for four months. She is also an author for the popular series *The Complete Idiot's Guides*, for which she has contributed nine books on topics ranging from cooking substitutions and fondues to smoothies and fast and fresh meals.

Ellen's writing has appeared in more than two dozen publications, including the *Washington Post*, the *Los Angeles Times*, *Bon Appetit*, *Art Culinaire*, *Texas Monthly*, *The Baltimore Sun*, and the *San Francisco Chronicle*.

Honored by *Cook's Illustrated* in the prestigious "Who's Who of Cooking in America," Ellen has been profiled in *The Washington Post*, *The Detroit News*, *Coastal Living*, and *The Miami Herald*.

She lives in Providence, Rhode Island.

Karen Konopelski, M.S., R.D., is a nutrition consultant at Princeton University. A former sports nutritionist at the University of Connecticut, Karen's work experience includes providing one-on-one counseling to athletes on issues ranging from nutrient timing and eating-to-perform to eating disorders and weight loss. She has also worked at the National Institutes of Health in Bethesda, Maryland.

Karen received her certification in dietetics from New York University. She lives in Princeton, New Jersey.

INDEX

Note: Page numbers in italics indicate photographs.